Silvia Buffagni (Esperide Ananas),
SPIRALS OF ENERGY, The Ancient Art of Selfica

Translation: Quaglia (Juliette Chi)

Editing: Esperide Ananas, Gwendolyn Grace

Photos: Gianluca Scolaro, Esperide Ananas

Graphic design: Gambero Finocchio Selvatico

ISBN 9788890863714

Devodama srl, Vidracco (TO), Italy

With many thanks to Gwendolyn Grace for her support and generosity that made the English version of this book possible.

Esperide Ananas

Spirals
of Energy

The Ancient Art of Selfica

To Falco

Introduction

In this book, Esperide Ananas tells about her experiences with Selfica and introduces many other researchers, both Damanhurians and non, who over time have established a strong relationship with these particular energetic-intelligent structures. She begins with Falco of course, who is the inspiration for Damanhur, Federation of Communities, and who presented Selfica in the mid-seventies.

These research experiences are often conducted with considerably complex Selfic devices, which are found alongside the selfs for daily use such as those that are available to everyone at the SelEt studio in Damanhur Crea.

A few centuries ago, writing a book like this would have been a shortcut to the stake. Until a few years ago, it would have been a source of ridicule for the author and those sharing their stories, in the name of common sense which—regardless of what you really think—labels experiences related to sensitivity and sensibility as superstitions. However, times have changed, and now it is not so strange to talk about the universe as energy shaped by thought, and experiences at the border of science and spirituality such as those told in this book have space and attention.

Quantum Physics opens perspectives on time and space that are not only mechanistic. Through psycho-neuroendocrinology, medical science attests that positive thinking improves and extends life. Multidisciplinary researchers at the crossroads between science, philosophy and poetry, delineate the pathways for exploration of life.

In this vein, we find Selfica, a discipline that departs from a two or three-dimensional physical object—copper bracelets, larger installations, paintings of different sizes—and makes it so that the object can host a purely energetic intelligence that exchanges information with the person who owns it. In this sense, the selfs and Selfic paintings can be considered living objects that exchange energy with their owners—energy directed toward the wellbeing, equilibrium and regeneration of the person.

Selfica is a research discipline that originates from ancient knowledge recuperated from the depths of time, located on the imaginary library shelves that contain the knowledge of all humanity, and brings this knowledge together with patient experimentation. For nearly forty years, Falco himself carried out this research; many Damanhurians have helped him, some as the direct creators of various Selfic models, others simply as experimenters who use the selfs in everyday life. As with every Damanhurian discipline, in Selfica, experimentation is always carried out in the field. It is done "live" because the idea is not to fill tables with data and numbers—which is impossible in fields based on the direct empathy between a person and the phenomenon—rather, it is to discover each person's potentials and limitations and then push them a little further. For this reason, this book tells about experiences, emotions and discoveries that describe the relationship between humans and selfs.

Those who love science fiction can imagine this connection between the physical object and the energetic intelligence that "inhabits" it as the landing of a friendly extraterrestrial species, of intelligences that come from a different dimension with respect to ours. More simply, it is one of the manifestations of the spiritual ecosystem of our world.

Many living beings coexist in this ecosystem: beings who are conscious and self-aware, even in the absence of a physical vehicle. For example, there are devas who live in nature, great stellar forces, invisible helpers, and all of the larger and smaller forces that human sensitivity has identified and the imagination has described, according to different myths and traditions.

When the first models of selfs were developed, Damanhurians and friends acquired them in the spirit of using a natural and noninvasive method to increase wellbeing, balance one's own energies, and strengthen defense against external agents. Over time, our relationship with the selfs has changed. They continue to shower their benefits on those who use them, but the fundamental experience for many is the creation of a living space that is an extension of themselves and their own awareness. It is a new ecosystem, a natural habitat in which people interact with the selfs that have been around them over the years, from bracelets to jewelry and paintings. In this sense, the research is open and more expansive than ever...

Stambecco Pesco

Introduction by the Author

This book is a collection of my personal experiences and those of many others who tell their stories. They are episodes of subjective research and do not presume to be absolute truths. At first, I thought writing about Selfica was a task beyond my abilities; then, thanks to everyone's contributions, I believe this book can be useful to better understand one of the most fascinating aspects of Damanhurian research. Selfica, like any path of investigation at Damanhur, is always a shared endeavor, because the uniqueness of all those who contribute to it makes the end result more valuable and profound.

Selfica was introduced to Damanhur through Falco's studies. At the beginning of this book, an interview with Falco in the Spring of 2012 is transcribed and gives a basic introduction to what Selfic intelligences (or "selfs," as we normally call them) are. In the pages that follow, many Damanhurians tell about their adventures exploring a clear and constant channel of communication with these "intelligent energies," or border forces whom many of us at Damanhur have started to know over the years. Many principles of Damanhurian philosophy are also presented so that these experiences can be fully understood.

During my many years of experimentation, I have lived very exciting moments, as well as periods in which I felt I was a bit "dull." In the moments of unclarity, I needed to find a new centeredness and inner order so that I could reach the next level. The glimpses of awareness that the selfs have offered me and my fellow researchers have deeply changed our lives. These moments helped us to gradually open to a different and more articulated understanding of reality during a constant journey of heart and mind expansion. For this, I am deeply grateful to Damanhur.

I hope this book inspires others to embark with happiness and love on the most exciting adventure there is: seeking your place in the universe and collectively participating in the reawakening of human beings as a divine, material and spiritual principle. Now is the time.

Damanhur offers tools that everyone can use. In our philosophical school, we train to become "lucid mediums" of ourselves, of our own personalities, and of different levels of intelligences and forces. This means learning to be present in the linear time where we are, and with a part of ourselves being able to move beyond the customary cause-effect relationship. In this way, we acquire a method for "sensing" reality in a more expanded way. Selfs have revealed themselves to be exceptional, loving and tireless teachers... rich in a sense of humor! I imagine humor is an essential ingredient for them to collaborate with the human species, so often lazy, stuck in its habits, and also somewhat arrogant...

The experiments with the selfs call on us to welcome new experiences and ways of thinking, without judgment; at the same time, they teach us not to glorify ourselves through our revelations as if we have understood everything. Instead, every experience brings about more questions, fewer certainties, and a new desire for more explorations. The thousands of daily activities are an invaluable help for maintaining a healthy sense of belonging to this world, even when parts of us are involved in galactic explorations.

Life at Damanhur is full of experiences that are out of the ordinary. Our minds are constantly stimulated to open up to new possibilities and new understandings of every aspect of life, beyond appearances. We are people with our feet on the ground. We reconcile science fiction and research with personal relationships, children, work, study, agriculture... constantly reminding ourselves that our spiritual achievements are instruments for transforming material reality, in service to others for the awakening of humankind.

Section One

"CLASSIC" SELFICA

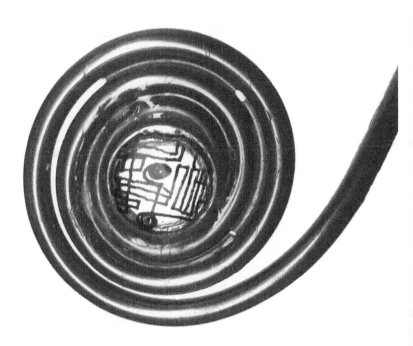

... it was a small spiraling copper structure ... it looked like a sculpture... even though it was simple, it had harmonious proportions, and the coils, which tightened horizontally until they came to a point with a single copper wire, seemed like it was actually creating a direction...

The first encounter

The first time I saw a "self," I was profoundly captured; a small spiraling copper structure placed on a shelf amongst books, medallions and a plethora of other objects, and it stood out to me as though a spotlight was shining on it. The identification card said that it was an "environmental balancer," built to keep the atmosphere of a space energetically "clean"; its function was to direct to the outdoors any traces of disharmony so that they could dissolve back into nature. The self looked like a sculpture. Even though it was simple, it had harmonious proportions, and the coils, which tightened horizontally until they came to a point with a single copper wire, seemed like it was actually creating a direction—the direction where, I imagined, the self was to invite stale thoughts to go out the door...

It was 1991, my first visit to Damanhur. I had come from Milan where I worked as an independent communication consultant, and my world was extremely different from that of a valley in the foothills of the Piedmont Alps. I had been drawn to Damanhur by a flyer I had seen in a friend's home, and my intention was to visit and dedicate only a few of hours of my time to the exploration of this rather unusual community... a few hours that have now become over twenty years.

I arrived at an unpaved parking lot, and there was hardly anything there except many trees, and the columns of the Open Temple stretching up to the sky, a stone spiral and small altars dedicated to the elements—simple but captivating, so much so that they seemed to emerge from a fairy tale book. People were relaxed, smiling and dressed in a way that seemed unusual to me. Many wore clothes made of handmade textiles and donned particular jewelry and ornaments, often made of copper with spiral forms similar to the object that had caught my attention. It was a bit like a cross between "The Lord of the Rings" and an ancient civilization that I could not identify. (Or maybe was it a civilization from the future? I wonder if the director of "The Green Beautiful"[1] was inspired by Damanhur. If the film had already existed at that time, maybe I would have placed Damanhurians in a very advanced galactic civilization.)

At the time, the Temples of Humankind were a well-kept secret[2]. The community presented itself as a spiritual center based

1. In 1996, the French actress and director Coline Serreau shot the film "La Belle Verte" (released in English under the title "The Beautiful Green"). On a planet far away and unknown to earthlings, humans live in harmony with themselves and with nature. After passing through the industrial era and experiencing its cruelty and horrors, they chose to break down hierarchies, factories, and everything that was part of an era of exploiting others and the planet. One of these evolved humans chooses to go on a mission to Earth …

2. After the first excavations began in the summer of 1978, the Temples of Humankind remained a secret for sixteen years. Only the Damanhurian artists, craftspeople and masons directly involved in the construction knew about it. Even though the Temples were on Damanhurian property, they were unauthorized because in the Piedmont region of Italy, there were neither laws that regulated underground construction nor authorities for the asking of permission.
In 1992, a former member of Damanhur sent an anonymous letter to the local police station affirming the existence of the hidden Temples. Armed and accompanied by explosive experts, the police came to the house where the entrance to the Temples were located on July 3, 1992 at seven o'clock in the morning. Oberto Airaudi, the founder of Damanhur, and Cormorano Sicomoro, one of Damanhur's lawyers, led the District Attorney of Ivrea and three police officers into the Temples. A fourth person followed them inside with a camera to film the visit. An hour later, the men came out of the mountains, and they were deeply moved and touched by the beauty of what they saw as the first witnesses from outside of Damanhur to see the Temples. On October 9, 1992, Damanhur held the first press conference to announce the existence of the Temples of Humankind, and the next evening, images of the Temples were transmitted in an exclusive broadcast on national TV. In June 1996, the existence of the Temples was legalized.
Excerpt from: *The Temples of Humankind,* by Esperide Ananas, Val Ra Damanhur 2006.

on natural medicine and the ecology of nature, thought and energies.

For Damanhur, those were years of developing a strong cultural identity; they were seeking a fully natural way of living, in contrast to the ways of the "external" world which was really consumerist at the time. A model of Arcadian pastoral harmony infused with eclectic and syncretistic spirituality? It was not so easy to understand at the time. The depth of Damanhur's message, without experiencing the beauty of the Temples, was only for those who could already sense beyond the veils of ordinary reality.

Luckily for me—ready to return to my beloved city without giving Damanhur a second look—there were the "selfs." I was intrigued because they seemed to be an incongruous element in that community lost amidst the mountains of a valley no one knew of at the time. They were a touch of sci-fi that made Damanhur very fascinating to me. I could not confine it within the definition of an "ecological community," something that in those years, did not attract me at all.

So, I bought that environmental balancer for my home, as well as a gold bracelet that was supposed to "harmonize my aura." The function seemed interesting enough, but most of all, the jewelry was beautiful. The gold coils gave it a characteristic style that I had never seen before, and yet it seemed familiar. And if I let it bounce between my fingers, it made a perfect jingling sound, as if it were a small bell.

I was told that these were not mere objects, but instruments able to catalyze energies and perform a specific function, determined by the shape, quantity and size of their coils. The materials with which the selfs were constructed also played an important role because each metal has a specific conductivity that determines which structure is to be created.

Somewhere deep in myself, all this sounded not only possible, but also somewhat familiar, something I already knew. Metals that could become "alive," so much so that they could be a support for intelligences that normally do not interact with our space-time... Precisely because of this, they are capable of acting on the border of the laws of physics, making experiments possible, combining mind, sensitivity and technology. Structures and machines that are alive? It was clear that the very idea of technology at Damanhur was totally different from the mainstream worldview in those years.

Today, little by little, more recent theories are coming closer to the theoretical-practical framework offered by Damanhurian Spiritual Physics, the discipline that researches the laws of our universe and of time, combining them with the meaning of human existence in the world of forms. The most recent treatises on physics and cosmology often seem to be mystical texts, and recent scientific discoveries are gradually leading to a transformation of the dominant paradigm. Optimists by conviction and choice, we Damanhurians hope there will soon be a generation of established scientists, no longer limited by religious or materialistic prejudices, capable of conducting research with a holistic—and therefore sustainable—vision of human beings and its relationship with the universe. In the early nineties, however, the terms of quantum physics that have become so common today didn't even exist in the common vocabulary.

I asked some Damanhurians how they came to these understandings, and to the development of Selfica. I was told that the foundations of this discipline were part of the memories of Damanhur's founder, Oberto Airaudi, Falco.[3]

Over the years, other researchers had been joining him, to continue this investigation in the field of energy combined with the use of metals. They told me that Selfica is an ancient art that creates structures based on a precise mathematics, able to connect

---

3. Oberto Airaudi (1950-2013) is Damanhur's Spiritual Guide. In accordance with the Damanhurian tradition of adopting animal names, he also used the name "Falco" (Falcon).

Falco was a philosopher, healer, writer and painter. He was continuously involved with research into cutting-edge therapeutic techniques, the Arts and New Sciences. From a very early age, Falco manifested a clear spiritual vision and the gift of healing. He was committed to developing them through constant and exacting experimentation, outside of traditional academic institutions. His spiritual and personal growth continued over the years through incessant studies, research journeys, reawakening of memories, development of artistic skills and rediscovery of ancient knowledge. In 1975, he founded the Horus Center in Turin to present the outcome of his research and initiate a more intense phase of shared experimentation. It was the first seed for a Mystery School and a community. From these activities the spiritual and social experience of Damanhur, Federation of Communities, has developed.

At the core of Falco's vision is the belief that every human being has a divine nature to reawaken within oneself, through conscious interactions with others. His teachings encourage the awakening of the inner master within each one of us, through study, experimentation, the complete expression of individual potential, and overcoming dogmatic attitudes.

Falco's autobiographical account of how he began to experiment with Selfica and recover his memories and full awareness of the project of Damanhur can be found in the book "Tales of an Alchemist," Niatel Edizioni, 2011.

19

to specialized and intelligent energies, in order to interact with people and the environment for physical and mental well-being, inner research, deep memories...

The simpler selfs, such as those that I saw the Damanhurians wearing, were made of metal, mostly copper, and there were also more complex ones that combined metals with spheres containing alchemical liquids acting as transformers of energies. Others united precious metals and microcircuits made with inks, and were specifically prepared to perform very complex functions.

Alchemical liquids? Intelligent metals and energies? Obviously I understood almost nothing of what all this meant, but these concepts stirred my curiosity. They were stimulating and really outside of the box!

Most of all, I liked the selfs. They fascinated me as objects. I liked to have them around me and to wear them, and I began to experiment with them. I felt they changed something in the environment. The atmosphere became more alive, and also my sense of well being increased.

I noticed that the bracelets I wore more frequently changed their shape, and all in a very similar way: that is, they adapted themselves to my aura, to the form of my energy field. I was particularly struck by the "joy self," created to spread the frequencies of sunlight into the environment for a specific radius around itself. Often I found it slightly elongated and turned toward our star, just as if it were a plant growing toward the light! Certainly, this was not a simple object, and the world of possibilities that this opened in my mind and my heart made me happy and ever more curious to continue exploring.

Selfica according to Falco's teaching

Falco introduced Selfica to Damanhur as a field of empirical research through his studies. In his presentation of Selfica below, Falco explains how the history of this art-science, which concentrates and directs specific energies present in our universe, unfolds over the course of many millennia.

"The esoteric tradition explains that Selfica was found back in the time of mythical Atlantis, as well as in civilizations of our historical era: Egyptian, Etruscan, Celtic and ancient Minoan. However, it was always reserved for specific social classes: the priests and rulers.

Selfica is a science that is widespread throughout the universe, and its history on our planet begins with a fundamental cultural change: shifting from a vision of the universe as a place where everything happens because of divine intervention, to the understanding that there are other forces at par with human beings, which

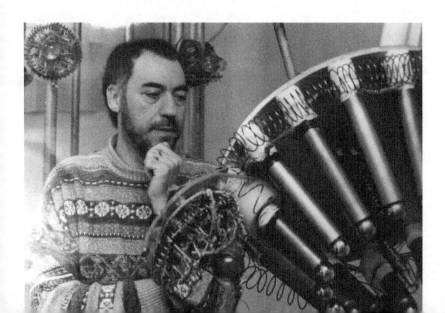

can be used to obtain the desired effects. Making sacrifices to a divinity was no longer necessary for a certain event to happen. Instead, it became necessary to explore what could be done by utilizing the forces of nature. Moving away from the idea of intervention from the gods to the idea that there are non-divine forces that are equal to or beneath human power who can produce the same effects, this was a huge leap in the way of thinking.

So, Selfica came about with this realization that there can be non-divine forces involved in changing events; it was a rationalization of magic. Selfica is a border science that goes beyond the pure and simple concept of magic, where the only way for anything to happen is by passively repeating rituals, and it introduces a creative phase in which human beings are active agents. As such, we can conceive of theories, create circuits, improve the system, establish the forces that flow within a circuit to a greater or lesser extent, in order to receive and direct these forces that exist in the universe. The forces are not just an interference with the field; they are a specific signal with qualities that we can use.

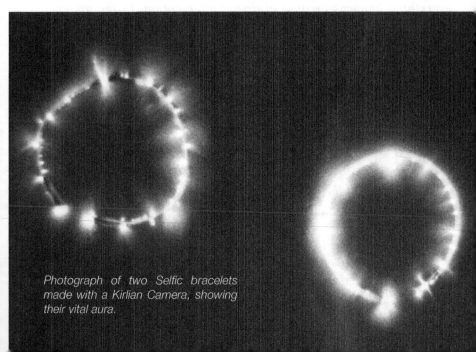

Photograph of two Selfic bracelets made with a Kirlian Camera, showing their vital aura.

In the distant past, priests were the first ones to notice the existence of these forces. They attempted to understand what kind of forces they were dealing with, learning to distinguish between the more important forces and the average ones. In fact, there are many intermediate measurements on a scale of value similar to the periodic table of the elements. Similar to this table, there are spectrums of forces that have to do with Selfica which include both intelligent forces—which we call as such because they respond in kind—as well as physical forces, which can be used to accomplish things.

All the efforts made through astrology were motivated by the search for these signals and frequencies, using different theories in order to interpret them. The intention was to be able to act upon these signals and not be limited by dependence on these universal forces, which are separate from human beings. However, astrology did not succeed in this step.

Ancient civilizations had also attempted to tap into these forces. In some eras, when the right metals and alloys for this purpose were not available, other systems were created using plants and especially water-based systems such as water labyrinths, irrigation and micro-irrigation circuits. With liquids, it is easier to interrupt the circuits, opening and closing them as needed.

Today, experimenting with and refining various aspects of Selfica has allowed us to develop what was not feasible in other times, because the right materials were not available then. Research in Selfica involves constantly expanding on the basic systems with different materials, which are sometimes more effective than the traditional ones.

In the past, gold and silver were the primary materials. By changing the percentage of copper or silver in the gold, differences in conductivity were created, although if you didn't know about this, you couldn't distinguish between the different potential of conductivity. In Damanhur, we often use copper for Selfica and mainly *inks, obtaining the same results with structures that are becoming ever smaller. We are now making structures that are able to receive, transform and use this signal to interact with synchronicity in an active way, aligning elements beyond simple probability, so it is possible to interact with the flow of events. 4*

Selfica allows us to receive the specific signals and the force, intelligence and energy that are needed for developing a capacity to shift the "containers" of events that we are constantly moving through. These containers are the ones that we intercept on different planes of reality.

4. Here is a brief description of Synchronicity and Complexity according to Damanhurian Spiritual Physics:

Synchronicity: is a force that creates a constant connection between all events, both simultaneously and along the line of time. So, the force of Synchronicity is the law that selects the events that occur at every point of space-time, surpassing the principle of cause and effect that is usually used to make sense of reality. From an individual point of view, we may encounter synchronic events, that is, events that have a positive effect on our lives, and asynchronic ones which are harmful to us. From the point of view of the universe as a whole, events are always synchronic and moving toward a common goal, which the Damanhurian school of thought identifies as the concept of Complexity. Synchronicity is not uniformly diffused throughout all of space-time.

Complexity: is the general direction in which all the forms of the universe are moving at different speeds. Complexity is also the goal of the universe itself, so we can say that synchronicity selects suitable events at the right time and place in order for the universe to produce Complexity. So, Complexity is the result of the relationship, the interaction between forms, of information exchange, in both quantitative and qualitative terms. Complexity is the element through which evolution occurs. According to the Damanhurian School, along the pathway of matter moving toward Complexity, there are four fundamental stages: non-life, life, thought and divinity—that is, absolute information at zero mass. Beyond this level, we find ourselves outside the universe of forms, in a new definition of existence that is still unexplored.

From "Esoteric Physics," by Coyote Cardo, Edizioni della Scuola di Meditazione di Damanhur, printed for private use, October 2009

The Selfic intelligences are more used to being in an environment where only energies exits, one that is beyond the material world. It is easier for them to act directly on the laws that maintain the universe in its field of existence, rather than on forms. As such, they experience a kind of linearity of existence that is very different from ours. We live in a three-dimensional world. One of the qualities of this world of forms is that it works through oppositions: black and white, heat and cold, dark and light... We transform this opposition into evolution, into change, because we begin with raw material and we modify it. This process is a part of spiritual refinement, a characteristic of living beings in this universe.

In their dimension, the selfs do not have the issue of opposition or the need to mature as we do, because in other parts of the universe, time is different from what it is here. In those places where the selfs come from, there is no flow of time as we can imagine it, so the forms or intelligences that inhabit it have different characteristics. Even though our concept of evolution cannot be compared with what happens in other parts of the universe, the extraordinary characteristic about these intelligences is that, in some cases, they are willing and able to connect themselves here and participate in our world, becoming symbiotic elements.

The Selfic intelligences and the humans who use them do not reciprocally interact in all aspects of life, but only for the specific ones where there is a mutual benefit. This symbiosis can be considered a true spiritual alliance between the selfs and humans. Selfs are interested in coming into the sector of the universe that is characterized by form, which is a part of the whole, and it allows them to be present in a different field of evolution. They can do this by connecting to ever more complex forms, such as the ones developed in current Selfica research at Damanhur. Today, thanks to this constant experimentation, Selfica can express itself in a multitude of supports, from metal objects to circuits made of inks and alchemical liquids, from paintings to gold and silver jewelry. The goal of the most evolved Selfic intelligences is to help human beings get closer and closer to their spiritual dimension. Humans are "bridge forms" between the spiritual and the material planes, a key connection point between matter and the subtle dimensions. There are other beings who are as intelligent as we are, if not more so. We are not at the top of the evolutionary ladder, but rather in an intermediate condition. So it depends on the choice of every individual, if we are closer to the forms that are beneath us, or if we can move our lives in a direction of spiritual choice, getting closer to superior forms.

In a system interacting with Selfic structures, that which transmits also receives. Just as there is a descendant effect, there is also an ascendant one. It's like a television that captures an image and transforms it into a specific signal, and at the same time, uses a camera to see how the audience reacts to the show and sends this signal back. In this sense, the idea that the selfs are having an experience in our space-time is valid, because the interaction is active and there are always interpretations, depending on each person's way of being. These interpretations are all valid, they just depend on the preparation of the person using Selfica. Some may interpret this interaction as love and growth.

In terms of their experience, there are selfs who are certainly more fortunate and encounter people who are more sensitive. This information is transmitted to every other Selfica structure, because the Selfic network is a real ecosystem in which every element is connected to the others."

The arrival of the signal

The arrival of the signal from the universal energies that Falco mentioned in the previous section, which allowed for the creation of Selfic transceiver structures, was not unexpected. It had been previously "announced" by the forces of nature with whom the first inhabitants of Damanhur had established a constant dialogue.

Orango Riso—one of the first citizens of the community and currently the Director of the School for Spiritual Healers in Damanhur, with a background in Computer Science and Cybernetics—tells how his history with the Selfic energies began even before the selfs existed in their present form. This happened when he and other Damanhurians were creating the community and coming into contact with the elemental spirits for the first time.

"I have always been very interested in developing my mediumship abilities, even before Damanhur was founded. With fellow researchers at the Horus Center in Turin, I was exploring extrasensory perception, in particular using the Ouiji board system with an organized group that met regularly. When we went to live in the first nucleo community, we realized that nature all around us was alive and present, and we immediately made attempts to contact these natural forces. What struck us right away, letting us know that we were really contacting them, was the fact that the messages we received spoke of our everyday lives, instead of talking about grand systems and abstract ideals, as is almost always the case when contacting "entities" on the subtle planes.

These elemental nature beings read our minds and our souls and interpreted what was happening during our days. They followed the sequence of events in our lives for a whole year, offering us interpretations, announcing events a few hours before they would

*happen, giving practical suggestions and leaving nothing to chance.
They did this in order to help us understand how much their subtle
world was linked to ours. They did experiments with us, "preparing"
seeds that gave rise to seedlings which were much more vital and
productive than the ones they hadn't treated.*

*We realized that there were hundreds of forces all around us
and that the transcendent world was one with the everyday world,
and one is the constant consequence of the other. When these worlds
are integrated, they exalt each other's complexity. For me, this was a
real consciousness awakening, because it not only explained things
and gave new meaning to my life, it also taught me how to read reality in a synchronic way.*

*These nature spirits described the richness of their world in this
particular point of time and space with great detail, explaining how
it all worked. We realized that the very survival of the world of the
subtle nature forces depended on our material world, on our actions, thoughts, and even the language we use. They told us that they
perceive everything in a synesthetic way; for them, smell, taste, color,
scent and sound are the same thing[5].*

*Profanity and aggression are destructive to them because they
"char" a part of the vibrational field, while harmonious and melodic
language attracts them as if it were a fragrant aroma. Also, a body
that is weighted down by excess food and alcohol emanates an unple-
asant vibration that they can clearly perceive, and it repels them. Just
as dirty and neglected places are unbearable to them. They told us,
"If you are present in yourself and in harmony with your body and
with others, you can create fruits that nourish our subtle world. If
you grow, we can grow, and we can serve nature better."*

5. During those years at Damanhur, an entire therapeutic study based on vibrational healing was developed, which involved "phono-chromo-therapy" sessions
in which sound and color frequencies are combined for a specific time period in
order to bring the body back to a state of optimal well being.

We understood more about the importance of creating a clean and harmonious spiritual "greenhouse." [6] *They said that this would also be essential for preparing a landing place for new forces, ones who were simple at first and who would become more complex—the world of Selfica was beginning to develop.*

6. The effort to create a spiritual greenhouse in which all life forms—the subtle ones from nature, animals, plants, humans and divine forces—are in harmony within an integrated ecosystem based on the richness of diversity is reflected in the behaviors, practices, and rituals of Damanhurians.

The Constitution states that *"Each citizen makes a commitment to spread positive and harmonious thought, and to direct every thought and action towards spiritual growth..."* (Article 2) and that *"Every Citizen lives in communion with nature and the subtle forces which inhabit it. Everyone is committed to respect and preserve resources, and to avoid as far as possible forms of pollution and waste."* (Article 6)

Also: *"Citizens respect their own bodies, taking care of them and nourishing them harmoniously, refraining from any form of substance abuse. They ensure the orderliness and cleanliness of their environment."* (Article 6) *"Every citizen is expected to be capable of self-control, purity in thought and action, and making mature choices."* (Article 3)

At Damanhur, we pay a lot of attention to ecology, energy with low environmental impact, keeping water clean, organic agriculture and alternative therapies. The lands of the community are clean, well-maintained and enriched with works of art. Citizens are always working to create more beautiful and welcoming spaces, taking care of the outdoor environments with respect for the history and topography of the area. For many years, the community has invested considerable resources in restoring a large wooded area that was damaged by decades of exploitation for the use of wood. Gradually, many animal species, especially butterflies and birds, are returning to inhabit this area.

In the central area of Damanhur called Damjl, the Woods of Consciousness is a protected space dedicated to Nature Spirits. Citizens only enter into this space for meditation or contacting these forces, which happens in a ritual way every Sunday. Also, Damanhurians have sealed an alliance with the Nature Spirits, in order to establish a relationship based on mutual attention, respect and cooperation. We remember and honor Nature Spirits during the great rites of the Solstices and Equinoxes. During these rites, as humans we affirm our awareness of being part of a great cosmic cycle where nature and its forces play a fundamental role for our lives and evolution.

They explained that the selfs were like bodies for attracting more complex beings, ones who are able to go beyond the boundaries of the astral world, where the nature spirits lived, and could interact with time in an expanded way. These forces were to become a bridge with "the boundaries of time," because they could increase synchronic potential, "dilating" the moment in a way to embrace several branches of time, so we could make choices based on a greater number of possibilities.

The first self that was created was for protecting and strengthening the aura, a single copper wire with coils at the two ends. The next one was for protection against radioactivity, which we only wore a few hours a day. For me, wearing a self was like strengthening the contact with the elemental beings, and I realized that the voices that I had trained myself to hear were exalted.

Then, there were new ones, and I was amazed how they could be conveyed in these extremely simple selfs. Their prompting voices overlapped with my inner ones, and I always subjected them to little tests because I was afraid of losing myself in my imagination.

A typical test was asking how many clients I would receive in my pranatherapy studio the next day. Once they told me that there would be twelve cancellations, and I didn't believe it because I had never had so many before. It turned out that an unexpected public transportation strike began, and I had exactly that number of cancellations.

I remember how surprised I was when shortly after this, the memory self was created. It gave amazing results for headaches and sore throats. We tried putting it to our foreheads by chance... and *just like that, we found a therapeutic instrument that could easily be used by people.*

Something similar happened with the self against neck pain. By turning the active part of the cir-cuit onto the throat instead of the back of the neck, we discovered that it helps the thyroid.

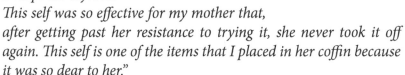

This self was so effective for my mother that, after getting past her resistance to trying it, she never took it off again. This self is one of the items that I placed in her coffin because it was so dear to her."

The personal Self

When I decided to go and live in Damanhur—I have been a resident citizen since 1993—there were already selfs for many functions, ones for personal use: for memory, for recuperating energy during sleep, for improving vision, for the aura and health, and there were also ones for collective use to harmonize the energies of the environment.

The most complex one was the "personal self," a structure that is specifically created for an individual with functions related to synchronicity and possible pathways of destiny, protection and memory, both in the present lifetime and after leaving the physical body.

Orango recalls, "*When personal selfs were created, there was a leap forward in complexity and sensitivity, because just as the nature spirits told us, every time new results were obtained in the field of Selfica, the logic of the whole system changed. For me, what changed was my way of feeling and intuiting in my healing profession and in my life, and my relationship with the complexity of my life was transformed. With my personal self, I experience a real and alive connection, as if this instrument were a new limb that activated new parts of myself of which I sensed the potential, but I did not yet have the full use. I had the same feeling years later when I began working with very complex selfs for healing work and dowsing to explore physical and mental wellbeing.*"

A personal self is the most complex Selfic instrument for individual use. This kind of self "lives" in symbiosis with the person using it. In this way, the individual chooses to establish a spiritual alliance with these kinds of forces. There is an extraordinary opportunity for evolution and experience at this crossing point between the human dimension and that of the personal self.

The selfs prefer being at the point where contrasts come together, such as in our species, because we have a material nature and we also host a divine principle.

From this perspective, according to Damanhurian research, the personal self can serve as a channel to establish a relationship with the divinity that each one of us has within. They can also help us to more effectively use a part of our dormant faculties, that are not normally available to us but are anyhow present in all human beings[7]. The personal self acts as a kind of "protective suit," as a buffer space for the individual, since its purpose is to divert certain events and to direct others.

7. According to recent studies in neuroscience, adult human beings in this stage of evolution, although mechanically using 100% of the brain, only use a part of their cerebral faculties, and we are still very far from the ability to use both hemispheres of the brain simultaneously. Rare cases of people who are able to do so — spiritual teachers, great artists, yogis — demonstrate that everyone has this potential, but out of habit, culture and constraints, we are not able to activate this capacity.

Ninety-five percent of the functions of the human genome have not yet been discovered. In fact, only 5% of our DNA encodes the proteins that are then manifested in the phenotype of the body. With arrogance that is typical of the scientific establishment, considering what they do not understand as impossible or useless, in the 1970s this 95% of human DNA was called "junk DNA" and considered irrelevant to the goals of research. Today, some scientists have begun to study this DNA and have discovered that it could play a crucial role in the evolutionary history and lives of many organisms. For this reason, they propose calling it "noncoding DNA" instead. Many parts of this DNA are "ultraconserved," that is, they have not changed over millions of years and are identical in many organisms, even though these species are now only distantly related.

The selfs act on Synchronicity, the law which allows the equilibrium that sustains life to remain constant. Events can be positive or negative only when they are in relation to the individual user. The personal self does not change events, rather it selects them and directs their field of action so they can be interpreted and therefore have an influence in a synchronic way rather than an asynchronic way. A synchronic event is one that opens up new possibilities, even if it may seem like a challenge at the time. An asynchronic event, on the contrary, has the opposite qualities, even though it may seem to offer an easy situation. The mental attitude that the person may have can of course have an effect, because a self cannot override the free will of its human simbiont; every human being is always at the center of his or her own evolutionary path, through choice and directed will.

The events are selected around a person based on their physical, mental, psychological and cultural structure, considering the evolution of the individual and their choices. This is possible because human beings have a soul, a sacred dignity and divine origin, so it is part of human nature to participate in spiritual dimensions on many levels of what is possible and on several branches of time.

The beginning of the connection

When a person wears a personal self for the first time, it is as if the self were "born." It is in that moment that the personal self connects to the energetic structure of the person, through the correspondence between the human energy system and the circuitry that the self incorporated in the self. Each personal self contains a map of the Synchronic Lines—the energy lines that wrap around our planet and, passing through the sun, connect it to the universe—and the map of the "microlines." The microlines are the equivalent of the Synchronic Lines in every living being on planet Earth. The microlines are the basic energy structure, the matrix of belonging to this world, the preferential path for our vital and sexual energy flow. In order to activate its functions in symbiosis with a human being, the personal self connects to the microlines, and at the same time, it helps to keep this system "clean" and in balance.

So, the individual who wears a personal self serves as the fulcrum for the functioning of the self. The self is nourished by the debris of our vital energy, that is, those energies that would naturally be wasted during movement and thought, during our very existence. This creates a mutually beneficial ecosystem. If you lose a self or do not wear it anymore, the Selfic intelligence tends to leave its structure. When a person is informed about what a self can do and uses it with some degree of attention, the contact between the self and the person is accelerated and deepened. In the same way, the personal self increases its knowledge of the person over time.

The functions of the personal self are now concentrated in a few square centimeters of circuitry drawn with alchemical inks. The different layers of alchemical patterns have connection points between them, not only horizontally but also vertically. To understand this system, we can consider the analogy of the ancient science of pentacles. For example, the esoteric tradition says that the pentacle created by Cornelius Agrippa was a system used to transmit information by overlapping certain patterns, which could be interpreted according to a specific code and rhythm.

Initially, the personal selves were larger, although their composition, shape and size have evolved over time, as happens with all selves, allowing us to create smaller and lighter structures. The first selves still had parts with metal spirals in order to make grids for energetic flows.

Later on, the atom concatenation was created in order to substitute the metal itself. "Concatenations"—another example of Damanhurian research in the field of energies from nature—offer the possibility of activating a specific and recognizable orientation in molecules, atoms and quarks inside a mass of any kind. This makes it possible to "draw" Selfic circuits inside of it, creating a sort of fabric or building conductors. This technology also makes it possible to create geometries suitable for making Selfic systems that can be programmed in multiple ways… ever more sci-fi!

A later and more refined system uses patterns made with alchemical inks. The inks are separated by thin films, because they touch each other only where it is needed. This creates a space made by overlapping layers and allows the circuits to be used, not only with a horizontal composition but also a vertical one.

A personal self created with microcircuits can be "housed" in an earring, a ring, a pendant, a small metal box... any object that is easy and comfortable to wear and that can have multiple layers of circuits within it. Personal self containers made of gold or silver also act as support for the memory of the self, which is "engraved" into the atomic structure of the metal.

A recent development in this technology is the "recall" (ri-chiamo) for the functions of a personal self. This is circuit of connections that allows you to leave the "main body" of the personal self in a safe place, so you do not risk loosing it, keeping the points of access and exchange within your aura.

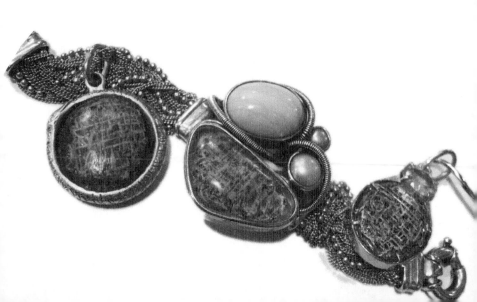

Establishing a relationship

The most interesting part of Selfica research is that it is based on a relationship with intelligent energies that can even have an emotional dimension established by both sides—the self and the person using it. Everyone who has a personal self or other Selfic devices with sufficient potential are constantly invited to experiment in many ways to create a channel of connection with these instruments and energies, one that is as very conscious and alive.

One of the many ways to deepen a relationship with your personal self is to discover its name, the sound-frequency which has an intrinsic relationship with an object/energy. Knowing the name of a personal self can help you to access its functions in a more conscious way. Even if you imagined or chose the name, it is still a sign that a relationship has been established, that there is a recognized code. A name can be a confidential element that facilitates a deeper exchange, as is the case for the names that we use as human beings.

Everyone has their own method for finding the name of a personal self. Sometimes it is easy to create the connection, other times it takes longer. I found my personal self's name quite easily by entering into a state of light hypnosis, which brought me into contact with the circuitry of the self, as if it were a book that I was lightly caressing with my thoughts. Then, I heard my voice say a rather long and very musical name very clearly.

Orango immediately received the name of his from the personal self itself. It was a confluence of names from other forces that he already knew, with some added endings. All the names are melodious, clear and modular, and they sum up the frequency of the selfs. Most people don't like to reveal this name because it is nice to keep it a secret, "just between me and the self."

Another way to find a personal self's name is to program a moment of "contact" in dreams, or to direct the mind in order to find it in a synchronic way. Antilope Verbena is one of the directors of the Damanhur University, as well as a professional nurse and healer with many years of experience in using Selfica for mind-body wellness. She discovered the name of her personal self by combining these two different methods.

"To deepen the relationship with my personal self, I wanted to find out its name right away. I thought about it a lot, but I just couldn't hook it. I knew that my self contained dreams I am to dream in this lifetime—recorded in the rose quartz, one of its components—so, I asked it to tell me its name in a dream. I dreamt of a book of fairies instead. Long ago, I had read the name of an undine in this book. I liked the name so much that for a while, before choosing the name Antilope, I wanted that fairy name for myself. I found the book and opened it with the personal self in my hand. It showed me exactly the page that described this fairy, so I understood that it was not my name but that of my personal self."

The personal self is an essential tool for every Damanhurian. The self integrates and supports much of the research and many of the ritual operations that we perform, as well as the relationship with the Divine Forces and those present in the Temples of Humankind on all levels.

Sirena Ninfea, head of Damanhur's School of Meditation and the Way of the Oracle, often uses Selfica for ritual functions and ones related to the magical dimension of Damanhur. Sirena shares that the first time she realized a self was not just a simple object was indeed in connection with her personal self.

"I felt as if I had a new companion, like something alive and present had joined me. Right away, I knew the name of my personal self, so we immediately had a close relationship. I don't have con-

versations with the self, but I do feel its presence, and when I don't have it with me, I feel incomplete. I enjoy 'being in the company' of the selfs.

The first physical structure of my personal self was a small sculpture contained in a silver box. It was not miniaturized like the current selfs are, and it was made of copper circuits, brass, mica, lead, ink and circuits drawn on paper. A few years ago, that self was stolen, but its essence, experience and memory have been recalled in the one I use now, which is miniaturized.

A personal self selects events, and I feel that I have had a synchronic selection for my pathway; I feel that I have been helped. Of course I am always the one who is choosing, but thanks to this synchronicity, I feel like I have given deeper meaning to the actions of my life.

In Damanhur, I feel like I am within a Selfic environment. I can perceive Selfic frequencies everywhere: in the Temples, on our lands, in the organic food store, in our homes... Damanhur is a magical and ritual 'Selfic greenhouse,' and it's like living in a special laboratory, which I like very much."

People who regularly use selfs often feel a familiarity with the specific energy field that they create. Modern science has demonstrated that every living being and every object in the universe emits and receives energy, entering into relationship with others and the environment in ways that can be positive—constructive interference, or detrimental to life and development—destructive interference. On a quantum level, atoms are not composed of physical particles but energy vortices in relation to one another. Everything that exists in the universe is interconnected within the same energy field.

In an environment where selfs are present, people often sense a particular harmony because there is a coherent and ordered energy field. We are able to perceive this field because at the base of matter, there is nothing material, but rather interactions between energies that are constantly in connection based on their resonance. According to this principle, a coherent field not only affects humans but all living beings who are interacting within it. One of the experiments now taking place uses Selfic structures to create an ordered environment in the areas where beehives are located in Damanhur. The goal is to reduce the disorientation of the bees— a sad phenomenon that is leading to a drastic reduction of their population on our planet.

Also, Selfic fields are used to support the growth of vegetables in the greenhouses and fields. To complete the cycle, a complex Selfic panel has been in place for years at the Damanhur grocery store "Tentaty."[8] This Selfic structure "fixes" the energetic structure of the products entering and exiting the store, which makes it possible for their vital energy to last longer. In this way, they keep their nutritional properties intact for a longer time than they normally would within a field of random energies.

8. The organic foods and products emporium "Tentaty" is located in via Baldissero 21 in Vidracco, in "Damanhur Crea" Center for the Arts, Research and Well-Being. www.tentaty,it

Protection

All Damanhurians and many of our friends have personal selfs. These "animated Swiss army knives"—to quote a metaphor that Falco used to emphasize their versatility regarding our existence within a flow of events—are all connected to each other, and they can guide synchronic flow where it is most useful while in continual conversation with each other. The events we are immersed in can then be selected and grouped according to the individual and collective potential we can cultivate and express for our evolution.

Potentially life-threatening accidents are some of the most evident situations where a personal self can intervene on the course of events. Damanhurians and friends have had experiences where they were involved in very dangerous situations and came away unscathed, while their personal selfs were completely destroyed or had a large hold in the center. In those cases, the Selfic intelligence "saved" them from the most serious damage, and in doing so, they self-destructed. Other times, the selfs communicate through dreams, clearly expressing doubts or risks about certain choices we are making.

Gorilla Eucalipto, a researcher who has participated for many years in advanced experimentation with the use of Selfic intelligences, tells this very particular anecdote in which his personal self helped him to avoid a severe accident.

"I have always been attracted by Selfic intelligences, so over the years, I have sought out close and intimate contact with them. I had a deep and personal relationship with my self right away, and I believe it has saved my life on several occasions. This is a true story that demonstrates this, as incredible as it may sound.

Many years ago on a very cold autumn evening, I had to make an urgent delivery to the town of Alba in the Cuneo province of Italy.

I climbed into a van that was full of merchandise and departed. I had to go about 150 kilometers to reach my destination, and the road was curvy, dangerous and covered with ice, but I was determined to arrive safely at the destination, which I did. I unloaded the van and about an hour later, I was on my way back.

Right after I got on the road again, the fog rolled in. In addition to the other difficult road conditions, the fog made those 150 kilometers really tough. It was already dark and I was tired. The visibility was reduced to just a few meters. I kept up my courage, speaking to my personal self with feeling and asking it to help me get home safe and sound.

The road was really terrible while driving through the Langhe area, which had curvy roads without lines demarcating the lanes, and no illumination, not even a lamplight! I felt tension all over my body and the adrenaline pumping.

I kept up a constant dialogue with my only traveling companion, the self, in order to stay on track and get home. There was no one else on the road... only fools made trips in those kinds of weather conditions. I wouldn't do it again, though I was already in the middle of the trip at that point.

I passed many hours like this, and when I was about fifteen kilometers from home, everything magically disappeared. The sky became clear without a trace of fog, as if I had just exited from the inferno. I breathed a sigh of relief and expressed so much gratitude to my friend the self—even though I didn't know that the worst was yet to come.

Reassured by the suddenly improved weather, my attention began to fade and fatigue set in heavily. It was still very cold, and I zipped up my windbreaker jacket because the heating in the truck had stopped working. I was still talking constantly with my companion the self, although because of my tiredness and the drop in tension, I fell asleep on a long, straight stretch of the road!

I'm not sure how long I was asleep, though at a certain point, I woke up all of a sudden because two hands sprang out from underneath the driver's seat and began to touch my sides...

Then, before my dazzled eyes, they pulled down the zipper of my jacket with a quick "zip" and then disappeared underneath the seat again.

I heard the self speaking in my head, "So, what were we talking about?" In that moment, I realized what could have happened and didn't! I had to stop because I felt an overwhelming tremor, which was my fear discharging itself. I got out of the van and walked a few laps around it before opening the door and checking that no one was underneath the seat. When I returned home, it was already three o'clock in the morning, and I was very happy to be alive!"

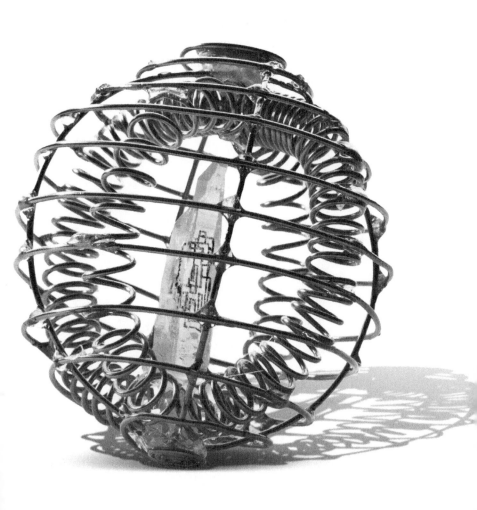

Individual explorations

Echidna Eufrasia is one of the researchers at Damanhur who is able to contact the selfs very easily. She has participated in many group experiments, and she also explores this contact with her personal self alone, which allows her to be guided in a more intimate research experience. She often uses her personal self to discharge tension, for self-healing, in telepathy experiments and to call upon characteristics that are useful in the moment. One of her most satisfying research experiences was a particular one she had with her plants.

"For a period of time, I got close to three seedlings that were in my room, using my personal self as a dousing pendulum. Each one of the plants had a very different personality, which at the time, I naturally associated with parts of myself. They communicated different preferences for begin watered and receiving light. I shared and exchanged emotions and feelings with them by contacting them with the self acting as an antenna. They each had different lives.

An event that struck me was that one of the plants, which I felt very connected with, was fine the day before, and the next day, it sacrificed itself. It had become black as if it were burned, after a powerful event that it had previously signaled to me. I think that during this contact, I established a real energy transference with the plant.

I sometimes ask my personal self to send me dreams, and the most beautiful one that came to me was about our planet, probably in the future. I was with others underneath a starry sky that was raining down an unusual golden-white powder. We were ecstatic because we knew that this substance had traveled through space-time dimensions to rejuvenate all of planet Gaia and its living beings. The surface waters and groundwaters were organically purified; the air

49

of the entire atmosphere of Earth was restored to its original pristine state; the vegetation transformed before our eyes, recreating itself in natural environments with enchanted gardens. In the human sphere, memories of illnesses such as cancer, abnormalities of the blood, and psychological disturbances, all just disappeared. Animal species corrected their forgotten course, rebalancing their seasonal cycles... everyone and everything was oriented toward the original equilibrium, a time when our earth was sound."

Ornitorinco Platano is one of the main researchers in the field of Damanhurian Spiritual Physics, and he is also an instructor for meditations and courses with the selfs. He says that his first contact with the world of Selfica was instinctive, and it later transformed into deeper research.

"From the beginning of my experience at Damanhur, I felt a strong attraction to Selfica. Even before becoming a resident citizen, I asked for information at the Selfica studio where they were created, and I ordered my personal self. Even though I didn't know exactly what it was, I felt a strong, instinctive call to have it.

My personal self was built on a gold ring with an eyelet filled with several layers of resin and ink circuits. According to the information I received during the public meetings on Spiritual Physics held every Thursday evening, these layers correspond to the specific operating codes for the basic laws in our field of reality. One of the many potential functions of a personal self is that it expands the funnel that events pass through, events that we are constantly attracting with our behaviors and thoughts. Because it has the matrix of the Law of Synchronicity inserted into its circuits, the personal self becomes a magnet for evolutionary events. It can amplify and select opportunities that are aligned with our choices and evolutionary path, harmonizing and extending the usual context we live in, thanks to the connection that all the selfs have amongst them.

It was 1994 at the time, and I was particularly enthusiastic about the topic of 'inner senses' i.e. our spiritual senses, and also experimentation with 'lucid dreaming,' where the Thursday evening lessons continued into the night.

We received appointments to meet each other in the 'Threshold,' one of the astral planes, or rather the intermediate state of non-time that surrounds our space-time. We used a special breathing technique and visualization of color-codes before falling asleep. It was fantastic to meet together in 'subtle classrooms' with the same people I attended classes with during the day. In this way, we could deepen our investigation and contact the energetic aspects of our knowledge about so-called reality.

During these lessons, we often took note of the deep feelings and emotions that could only be brought out in the Threshold. This gave us useful information for evaluating the state of our spiritual well-being, and how much we were able to draw from material experience, in terms of spiritual significance.

In normal conditions, the intermittency of our awareness makes it so that we can't easily conserve the 'substances' or emotional elements that are extremely important for nurturing the soul, our spiritual aspect. However, thanks to Selfic research, we were able to go much further.

I found study and research in these fields to be fascinating. Before coming to Damanhur, I had vaguely read about these topics in Carlos Castaneda's books, although at Damanhur, this kind of research was taken very seriously and also shared with others. To proceed with the research, I took exams to verify my preparedness and gain access to further phases of experimentation.

Some of these experiments required the use of advanced Selfic technologies, which at the time were inside the underground Temples, which I hadn't even seen yet. In those years, access to the Temples was reserved to Damanhurian citizens, and only in special ca-

ses for friends and visitors. So, it was through this passion of mine that I had the 'synchronic opportunity' to contact the Temples for the first time. From this point of view, I can say that my personal self has certainly worked by opening up this opportunity for me!"

Tapiro Acero since the beginning of the 1980s, has regularly participated in the "Viaggio," which means journey. The Viaggio is research and experimentation that Falco personally guided for many years, which involves traveling, sometimes great distances from Damanhur. Tapiro has a lot of experience working with Selfic energies, and he tells about his relationship with his personal self.

"I am a reserved person and not very emotional, but my personal self stimulates such strong and intense emotions in me. Very few things trigger my emotions in such an immediate way—only the stars perhaps, which I love to observe... For me, it is an instinctive gesture to pick up the small pendant that contains my personal self and talk with it and with myself, without distinction, expressing gratitude or sending a positive thought to the world, like the thought that humankind is succeeding in its reawakening, bringing the divine into matter.

In Damanhur, I am always conscious of living in an environment where Selfic energies are present, where they can be used for symbiotic support. They are so much a part of my life that I find it difficult to distinguish how using them increases my perceptive abilities. However, in some moments, my vision of reality was so different from those of others that I realized I have access to a different channel for using the senses, apparently mediated by the selfs.

One event that struck me happened at a place near Damanhur that used to be a sacred Celtic site. I was making love with my partner, and I perceived myself as a complex network of thin and very bright geometries. This network extended far beyond my head, as if I had an upper exoskeleton. This upper part made a deep impression on me. *I had a different understanding of how we are, or how we can be. I felt like I was not only living in a physical form of flesh and blood, but also as an extension made of circuits, energy lines, angles and velocity, just like that of the selfs.*

I feel a lot of love for my personal self because I sense that it is a being whom I know well. I get the feeling that I have been 'working' with it for several centuries, at least five or six, and that it has accompanied me in other lives. In this lifetime, it has been with me since 1986. Back then, I was living in the nucleo community where Falco lived as well. One evening when we were at dinner, he asked me all of a sudden, 'If you could ask for anything in this moment, what would it be?' I said the personal self. I had this very strong desire, and Falco gifted it to me. I felt like he was entrusting it to me.

I have traveled with Falco on Viaggio for 25 years, and in many moments, I used my personal self as a para-telepathic vehicle with him. Then, I began to think about other Damanhurians as well, trying to tap into their abilities, and I realized that it worked. I was one of the first ones to realize that there was this system of connection between us all, and I tried to understand how we could use it."

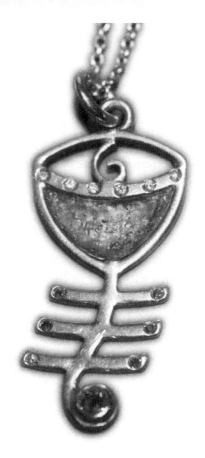

Temporary exchanges of characteristics...

As Tapiro described, we can use our personal selfs to connect with the characteristics of others who have one, in a kind of "para-telepathic" network that enriches all participants. This allows for a temporary transference of skills, so we can use the talents and knowledge of other people in this network whenever we need.

Damanhurians have experimented with these exchanges for many years, and some do so in a systematic way so they can be ready for anything. Antilope is one of them, and she has compiled a comprehensive list of skills that she lacks, identifying a Damanhurian that has each of these desired skills. It is a small, personal manual for emergency situations.

Antilope explains, "*I use my personal self a lot for para-telepathic contact, and I made a list of the people I know so I can access skills that I don't have when I need them. For example, I can use it when my car breaks down or if I need to change a tire, which really are paranormal events to me!*

This kind of exchange really works; it isn't just a result of suggestion, though I need to find people who are close to me in order to do it. Once I had to give a lecture in French, and I tried connecting with different people to improve my language skills in that moment. The first person spoke French as her native language, although I didn't feel like it was working. The second one was Italian, but this contact didn't work so well either. In the end, I focused on an Italian Damanhurian who grew up bilingual, and I felt my French was becoming more fluid and articulated. I think it's because, apart from the language itself, I had a closer relationship with her.

There was a funny episode a little while ago when I used this potential to get myself out of trouble. I was preparing dinner for three friends, and I really wanted to impress them. I'm not very good at cooking, though I had made elaborate preparations, and I was determined to make it work. Then, everything started to go wrong... it was almost time for the guests to arrive, and I didn't know what to do. So, I took some deep breaths and I thought about connecting with my friend Visone, who is an extraordinary chef. After a few minutes, I calmed down and everything started working perfectly. I was really fortunate because in Valchiusella, there aren't any take-out restaurants to use as a backup plan."

...and permanent ones

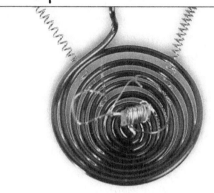

By using the personal selfs and the Selfic structures they are connected with, we can also have permanent exchanges of abilities. Tapiro was the protagonist in the very first experiment with this. He had a friend who was an expert helicopter pilot and had used many different selfs, someone who attended the Damanhur Center in Vercelli, Italy. Tapiro used a "copy" of this friend's ability to learn how to fly a helicopter. Even though Tapiro had already been attending classes to get a helicopter license, he learned with exceptional velocity.

"I participated in an experiment that was the first skill transference operation. Part of the reason why this situation was chosen was because we could have practical feedback to verify it right away. To avoid influencing the results, Falco didn't even tell me about this trial experiment at the beginning. Both of us enrolled in a helicopter pilot course.

Falco had transferred a copy of the skills from this helicopter pilot in Vercelli to me, while Falco himself started from zero. For a few days, I enjoyed a unique naturalness that allowed me to learn very quickly. I still remember the first trial runs for hovering over the ground, which is one of the most difficult maneuvers. After only an hour of practice, the instructor let me try it alone, and I was able to keep the helicopter in a very stable position.

After a few days, Falco told me that I was part of an experiment, and he asked me if I agreed to continue. I said yes, and I tried to figure out how to make the most of these characteristics. However, I realized that a mental approach didn't help; on the contrary, everything worked by letting things flow spontaneously, with amazement that then became energy that reentered in circulation."

Tapiro's instructors were astonished by his skills. They often said that he has an incredible knack for flying, as if he had always been doing it. Tapiro was very amused by these comments, although he let them go on believing in this innate talent instead of trying to explain the basics of Selfica on the takeoff field!

Language exchanges

The experiments for exchanging characteristics were also the first ones I directly participated in. In 1997, I lived with about ten other adults and three children at Porta del Sole, the house above the Temples, which was much smaller than it is now. The love and dedication we had for the Temples made us a close-knit group, and sometimes we were involved in special experiments.

With my friend Cicogna Giunco, I participated in a series of experiments for exchanging characteristics in the Selfic cabins. Discovering the characteristics of another human being is always an enriching journey that helps us to appreciate and love each other more, especially if I want to "insert" the qualities of another person within myself. Cicogna and I had established a deep connection between us and an energetic connection with the selfs. Cicogna is also the Damanhurian researcher with the most expertise in constructing selfs, and she has collaborated with Falco in this field for more than twenty years.

The operation for exchanging characteristics or acquired skills is very delicate, because each of these skills is accompanied by memories and emotions, which need to be harmonized within the alchemy of feelings and ways of thinking of the person who receives them.

The Selfic structure of the Temples worked as a "mediator" for the exchanges that Cicogna and I had, recording our aptitudes and finding the best way to harmoniously place them amongst the various parts of ourselves.

Like this, they could develop in an original way, a way that was consonant with the personalty of the person on the receiving end.[9] During the exchange, I had access to some elements of Cicogna's memories. I was particularly pleased to get some flashes from the years she lived by the sea, as she has always felt a deep connection with it.

Later on, I participated in another skill exchange experiment with Dugongo Canfora, a Damanhurian citizen who is originally Japanese. Dugongo needed to learn Italian very quickly in order to develop the Damanhur Embassy in her country. I know many foreign languages, and I can easily change my way of thinking according to the language I am speaking. These characteristics, along with the fact that I am a native Italian speaker, would help Dugongo to learn, offering her a predisposition which, along with her studies and dedication, would speed up achieving the desired results.

9. Just as the human body is comprised of many organs that create our physiological complexity, support for our mental complexity, including the soul, is made up of many parts that are recalled and ordered by a principle of divine intelligence. When integrated and harmonized, these parts—which in Damanhurian philosophy, we call the "personalities"—can reach a great spiritual complexity.

Every human body is the vehicle not only of a set of characteristics that are formed from the moment of conception onward, but also a "group" in which every component has a specific point of view, a "program" to carry out, a wealth of talents and memories. The part of us that comes into existence at the time of birth has a very important role, because it has the responsibility and potential for integrating all the others in a process of continuous expansion of awareness. However, it is not the only part of ourselves.

In Western culture, we are used to identifying with only one personality, whom we consider as "me," believing that it defines our uniqueness, and we really value our idea of personal identity. This "me," however, is not our complexity, but only a small and limited piece of who we really are. If we focus on just one aspect, we forget that every human being is a precious diamond with a thousand facets.

When I arrived at the Temples, I was feeling really excited, as I always do in these situations. I remember I was walking around and around in circles within the large, beautiful Selfic Cabin, which was located in the Hall of Water at the time.

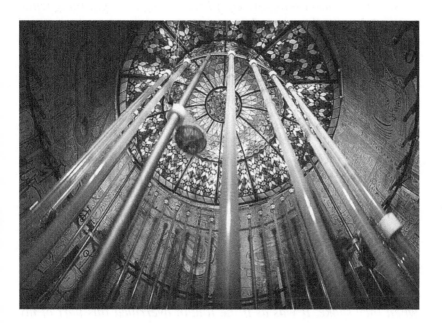

In addition to commonly used words, I was repeating all the Italian poetry that I knew from memory, parts from the Divine Comedy as well as contemporary poems, hoping that Dugongo—who was in the smaller Cabin next to the Hall of Spheres—would receive elegant vocabulary for expressing elevated concepts.

I was concentrating on the deep, ancient feeling of love for beauty and harmony that characterizes the Japanese people. I know that these exchanges are always equal and useful, and I am certain that my personal self is a precious reservoir of this experience as well.

Dugongo shared her impressions of this experience with me. *"I remember I was very excited and emotional. I was a bit intimidated by the fact that I was in a Cabin that had been used for many experiments related to time. I wondered if the exchange with Esperide would work for me, because I believe I'm a pretty 'hard-headed' person. I was also asking myself if I was doing the right thing while in the Cabin: walking in a clockwise circle with my thoughts focused on a particular kind of language exchange and on my state of mind in the moment.*

After what seemed like a long time, someone came to me and I got out of the Cabin. I discovered that it had been only fifteen minutes. I felt like nothing had happened, and I was a little disappointed...

I asked Falco if it had worked, as he was the one who coordinated the experiment, and he smiled and said not to worry because in the following days, I would start to see the evidence. In fact, I was able to learn a decent level of Italian in just two months, integrating the effects of the Cabin with effort and study. With this skill, I began developing the Damanhur Embassy in Japan.

There was a curious side effect for a while. I found it difficult to speak English, even though I could read and understand others when they spoke. It was as if the Italian overruled this part of my brain. Then, I realized I had not received Esperide's knowledge of the Italian language, but rather her capacity and flexibility in learning foreign languages. Fortunately, I regained my capacity to speak English later on.

Since I still had difficulty doing translation in public about the various topics of Damanhurian School of Thought, I also had help from a Selfic bracelet programed with the entire body of knowledge in the Italian language. With this, I was able to receive the meaning and understanding of words that I didn't know. It was an amazing experience."

Other Damanhurians have experimented with exchanging knowledge of foreign languages, with different and always interesting results. Sirena used the "copy" of another Damanhurian's ability in order to improve her fluency with the English language. What struck her the most was realizing that she acquired a different way of shaping her mouth, which allowed her to make the right sounds effortlessly.

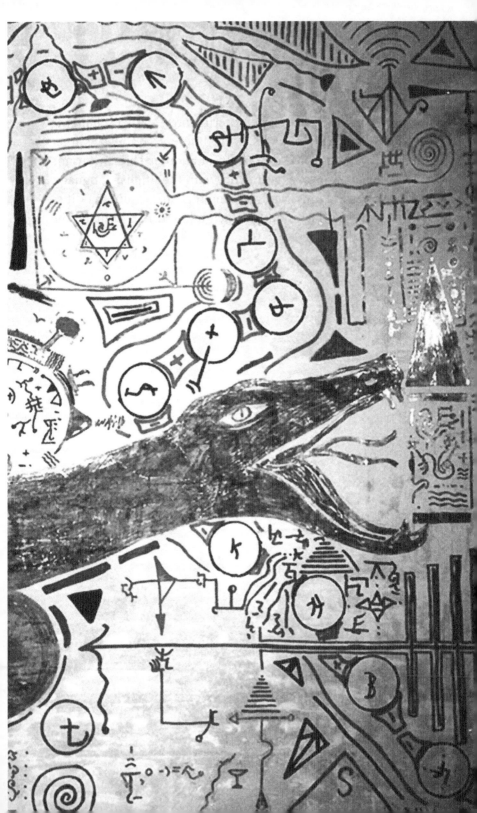

The Temples as a large Selfic structure

Many experiments with the selfs have been done in the Temples, because this underground complex contains the largest Selfic structure in the world. The Selfic structure transforms the Temples into a "living machine" that can open doors of communication with cosmic intelligences, receiving and sending signals and messages, and allowing for advanced experimentation—not easily explained by modern science—about the functions of time and the different potential levels of reality.

At Damanhur, nothing can be understood with just a linear vision, as our research moves toward ever more complexity and deeper meanings about our existence. Every "construction," whether it is physical, social, magical or spiritual, can be understood and appreciated only by integrating a multiplicity of perspectives and ways of thinking. By embracing many levels of understanding and expression, we can come closer to a relationship with reality that is not rooted in duality and opposition, but rather includes the many faces of what our philosophy calls the "crystal of truth."

The Temples are a prime example of this multiplicity of function and meaning. The various halls of the Temples are sacred spaces for contacting the divine, and at the same time, thanks to the relationship we have with higher forces, they are also a large laboratory for experimentation. These laboratories work when we use them as complete human beings, showing up with our emotional and sensitive sides as well as the analytical one, while practicing the "Art of Science," to quote Leonardo da Vinci. From our perspective, research should not be conducted in aseptic places, but rather ones where—given the condition that results can be measurable and if necessary, reproducible—everything within human beings can come to light, most of all the mystery, what is as of yet unknown.[10]

This is another reason why the halls of the Temples are extremely rich in various kinds of artwork, and the architecture also includes sounds and scents. The impact on our perceptions is so intense as to saturate the usual channels and "turn on" different ones in our minds, different ways of relating to the environment. Practically speaking, it is the opposite approach compared to the absence of stimuli in Eastern traditions, which achieves the same result. The result is that our mind is at peace, calming its constant chatter; the most profound parts of ourselves come to the surface; I am able to hear the voice of the soul, not only as a feeling of mystical transports, but as a non-localized field of infinite possibility which can be translated into concrete results in our space-time. The Selfic intelligences modulate and mediate these relationships, creating the intersection between human perception and our senses with the logics and mechanisms that transcend our conventional reality.

And my little conventional reality was completely transformed in January 1999.

10. A more modern citation of the same concept comes from Jonah Leher, a blogger and author of many books on creativity, intelligence and neuroscience. In "Proust Was A Neuroscientist," he writes: "We now know enough to know that we will never know everything. This is why we need art: it teaches us how to live with mystery. Only the artist can explore the ineffable without offering us an answer, for sometimes there is no answer. Keats realized that just because something can't be solved, or reduced into the laws of physics, doesn't mean it isn't real. When we venture beyond the edge of our knowledge, all we have is art."

Experiences in "Viaggio"

It was an intense period for the Journey, the "Viaggio." Falco was bringing different people with him for movements and experimentations in the big campers, to explore many fields of research on a deeper level. Communication with the selfs was amongst these areas of exploration. Until that time, our relationship with these intelligences had been more instinctive, based on sensitivity and intuition. Falco told us that in that moment, we could add a new dimension, a more direct communication with the selfs. We could open up a real dialog with them.

The Selfic structures had reached such a level of complexity that they were able to interact with our minds in a way in which we were completely conscious, using language and all the senses. "Second generation" selfs had been developed for a few years already. These are instruments that combined the metal components with spheres containing alchemical liquids, which had new and very articulate functions. These selfs were all connected to each other, despite the distances between one self and another. Connecting with one of them meant entering into contact with an intelligent and living network that extends all over the world.

When Tapiro Acero invited me to go with a group of experimenters who would join Falco in Viaggio the following weekend, I joyfully accepted. I could hardly wait for Saturday morning to come!

It had been almost two years since I had last gone on Viaggio, and I was looking forward to the pleasure of being in that "bubble" of special energy, where every thought and gesture resonates with unusual ways of thinking, where everything that happens can be used as a clue to discover new elements in research and understanding. Being in Viaggio means being the human component of a being of great complexity, who moves on many potential dimensions and levels. It's a kind of parallel reality that we participate in, giving meaning and direction to thanks to the alchemy of our attention, emotions, gestures and the relationship that we have with ourselves, others and the environment around us.

In addition to Falco and Tapiro, the crewmembers were: Quetzal, Raganella Lilium and Barracuda Tiarè. We moved in two large campers that were completely transformed into Selfic and alchemical laboratories. Falco used the one called "Arielvo," and we used the one called "Thor" as an experimentation field for those of us in Viaggio, called "Viaggiatori." Falco let us be completely free in choosing our research methods, which at the time were focused on finding a form of communication with the Selfic intelligences.

For this reason, we had an extremely complex Selfic structure in the camper with us. It was comprised of numerous spheroselfs, which are selfs that can be programmed for many uses, each with a liquid-filled sphere that amplifies the effects of thought. These spheroselfs were connected with each other in a circle, with crystals for programs, memories and many other Selfic connections.

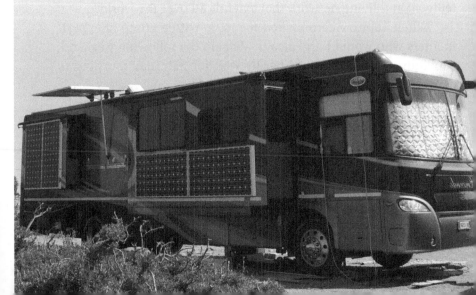

This Selfic structure was part of a larger structure that was still in Damanhur, and they were connected, despite the fact that they were separated from each other physically. The large Selfica "crown" was attached to a steel support structure that allowed us to move it, positioning it in the center of the camper table, as all of us sat around it in a circle.

Raganella had begun to sense a contact with this self through the dream dimension, and she had the impression that these intelligences were trying to understand the way we felt, in a mutual exchange with them. She had the sensation that unusual thoughts outside of the norm were coming to mind, and so she wanted the self itself to tell us about its potential use.

Previous groups had already achieved some decent results in connecting to the self through the use of dousing pendulums and other relaxation and hypnosis techniques, though we wanted to try a direct communication, a real "channeling" of the Selfic intelligences.

After doing a few minutes of deep breathing to tune in with ourselves and the others, together we projected our desire for contact with the self. I felt that we had made the connection right away… It is very difficult to use words to describe the sensation of becoming part of a larger energy, one with a different frequency than what the matter we are made of normally vibrates in. I felt dizzy as a light heatwave pervaded my body. I was a lucid observer, but a little bit off from my usual perception. I heard myself speaking, roughly at first, then ever more normally while the Selfic intelligences understood how to best use human physiology.

The self began to guide us in exercises to connect with one another, to create a united vibrational field comprised of everyone's characteristics. A deep sensation of peace and love pervaded us, while all of our colors became part of a single palette. We felt everyone's individual essence, but there was no more separation!

During those days in Viaggio, we performed many experiments and had many "contacts." In linear time, as measured by clocks, these experiments lasted about twenty minutes each, although our subjective perception of time was extremely variable. Sometimes it felt like it lasted just a few seconds, others times it seemed like hours had passed. With every experiment, the selfs guided us in new explorations, most of all in the unified field between us and with the different vibrations of matter.

We explored colors and substances, geographical locations and different spaces, perceiving everything in terms of geometries, angles and frequencies. Reality had become a field of relations and vibrations that we could codify and interpret with our sense perceptions and emotions. We felt that this was reawakening memories within our cells, like an awareness of belonging to a field of intelligence and love that gave meaning to our existence.

Raganella, who has been coordinator for the Viaggio for more than 15 years, has seen the "birth" and "growth" of many selfs, which the Viaggiatori have experimented with. The first one that she remembers is the one in which we had established a first contact with in those days.

She recalls, *"In 1998, Falco built this self, which we call the 'Concatenatore,' and as he usually does when he creates a new instrument, he told us to try and identify its uses. At the beginning, we didn't really know what to do, so we just observed it, hoping that some interesting inspiration would come to us. Even its presence in the camper created an energy that was like a waking dream, and we could feel our emotions in an amplified way.*

The selfs are beings that have an effect on emotions, and for me, contacting them is always very intense. In some experiences, we attempted to interrogate the self and have it tell us what its functions were. What was clear for us was that it worked with our mind states, leading us to emotional exchanges that were beautiful and very intense. Pleasant sensations and thoughts came to us in our minds, though it was difficult to codify them.

That weekend, Esperide was in Viaggio with us. She was able to get into a deeper contact with this being, and together we had a wonderful experience, a real journey through matter. It seemed like we were on a carousel of colors and shapes, and I felt like a drop within a drop of water, a spec of earth in the earth. I was able to feel the textures from the inside, as if I were a microbe, a bacteria. A truly exciting experience! What's even more amazing was that we were a group of five people, though each in our own way, we all had the same experience.

We experimented with the self in various ways, and we realized that after doing some breathing exercises and getting into contact, the self was working within us on a deep level, allowing us to explore new senses that weren't the usual ones on the physical plane. In fact, we discovered that this kind of self could help us to train in using our 'inner senses,' the subtle and profound senses. With this self, we continued doing many other experiments, and I realized that directing will power through the self works best if it is the result of a group instead of a single individual, if we use the sense of desire together."

On the drive back to Damanhur on a Tuesday, we parked the camper along the shore of a lake, and Falco said that we had time for a new exercise. We placed the self at the center of the table, held hands, breathed deeply, and off we went... All of a sudden, we found ourselves in the middle of the lake. It was as if we were the lake, which perceived itself through us. The structure of the water atoms danced before us as we sensed the connections. Suddenly, we heard a loud, deep sound that shook the lake from within, and the water molecules moved in a centrifugal direction, creating a vortex of energy that we perceived as a bright yellow color-frequency...

We immediately found ourselves seated at the table again, a little shaken up as if we has just finished a fast descent on a roller coaster! I felt like I was in a new world, like for the first time, I was beginning to feel how marvelous and alive everything was.

We got back to Damanhur in the late afternoon, after three days in Viaggio that had enriched us with knowledge and emotions which we couldn't have predicted before departure. As soon as I got down from the camper, I rushed to the Selfica studio to find Cicogna and share what I had discovered. Almost in unison we said, *"I don't know how to tell you about what happened to me this weekend!"* We looked at each other in amazement and began to share our stories, only to discover, with even more amazement, that we had the same experiences, particularly in the lake!

Sunday morning during a ritual in the Hall of Mirrors in the Temples, the sound of the gong had transported Cicogna beyond her normal perception, and she found herself underwater, sensing the molecules vibrating, moved by the force of the sound vibrations. So, that's where that loud sound had come from, the one we heard while in the camper... it certainly didn't come from us, it seemed.

The subtle and energetic connection between Cicogna and me, which had been established during our experiments with the cabins, had created an overlapping of reality, mixing parts of the events we were experiencing in different places. Since the selfs act in a way that is non-localized and not limited by an apparently linear time sequence, Cicogna's experience in the Temples Sunday morning corresponded with our exploration of the lake on Tuesday.

For us, this was a real epiphany that opened a space within us to a completely new reality, one that was not theoretical or limited to the great mystics, but something that we could understand and, we hoped, share with everyone else.

The Inner Senses Seminar

We began creating a pathway with successive steps that could become a seminar, an occasion to relive those experiences and open up to new ones. Damanhur is primarily a spiritual school, and the knowledge is not a set of ideas but rather a living element that can bring about a real transformation of that which is human to that which is divine. It is not an end in and of itself; it is an instrument to transform the self into Consciousness.

We sensed that the kind of perception the selfs were training us to use could bring us closer to the divine within us, because this perception transcends the everyday use of the senses, uniting heart and mind, opening space for new understandings, and leaving us with a mystical and profound sense of belonging to the whole.

The divine within each of us not only participates in our world as an observer, but if reawakened, it can become a co-creator. According to this point of view, at the dawn of known history when our species reached a sufficient physiological and neurological complexity, forces that were more evolved decided that we were a suitable species for hosting an active principle of transcendent awareness, a "divine spark." So with this perspective, we can harmonize the theory of evolution and the ideas of creationism.

This self-aware spiritual principle gives us the opportunity to serve as the "senses" of the divinities, who can have an experience in the world of forms through us, a world that they themselves created. So, the divine spark is the carrier of responsibility and free will, and it can help us to become conscious agents of the divinization of matter, that is, the extension of consciousness within the universe.

To reach this goal, it is essential not only to see, touch, hear, taste and smell the world around us, but also to transform our wavelength in order to become the "things" that we want to explore, to feel that they are really a part of us, that everything is connected in a profound and marvelous order, which we are separated from and which we can become aware of.

In order to do this, we need to awaken what at Damanhur we call the "inner senses," the senses of the soul. Through these sensory channels, we can explore communication with beings who are very different from us, like those conveyed by the Selfic structures, and we can also begin to contact and use the prerogatives of the divine parts of ourselves.[11]

11. The inner senses correspond to inner faculties, and they are a prerogative of beings who, like ourselves, consciously host an active divine principle. This divine aspect which is present in us makes us "bridge forms," structures of sufficient complexity that we can create a connection between the material plane and the spiritual one. As such, we are one of the forms on this planet able to operate as the senses of divinity, a combination of body and mind suitable for the experience of an absolute principle within the multiplicity of the universe of forms.

So, the "divine spark" allows us to develop the inner senses, and these sense make it possible to participate in a complete way in the natural and spiritual ecosystem that we are immersed in. We must guarantee the equilibrium of this ecosystem while it is in continuous transformation.

In these years of exploration, we have explored five inner senses in particular, which are defined as follows:
1. Sense of dream: the ability to perceive states of being, which are maintained without the necessity of form or the idea of form
2. Sense of desire: the quality of being able to direct one's own creative will
3. Sense of memory: the awareness of our contemporaneous existence in many points of time
4. Sense of exchange: the perception of and sharing in the meaning of other people's experiences
5. Sense of the divine: the awareness of our divine origins

In our research, we have also experienced a "transversal" inner sense, a support for the reawakening and integration of all the others: the "sense of love." This sense is the awareness of being part of an intelligent and sensitive whole, with an evolutionary purpose that goes beyond the single individual, the species and the planet. The full expression of our inner senses presupposes the integration of our personalities and using our vital energies in a correct and aware manner. Only in this way, it is possible to reawaken the divinity within each one of us.

So, we thought of creating a course called "Reawakening the Inner Senses," to explore how far the selfs could guide us in deeply contacting ourselves and expanding the perception of reality. At the time, we did not have much experience in conducting courses, but our enthusiasm seemed to be contagious. More than sixty people enrolled in the first course, and there were already six sessions planned for the future. All the Damanhurians who chose to participate were on board for a great adventure, for them as well as the instructors!

We defined a program, thinking about the ideal sequence of exercises. We chose music and various scents to stimulate the external senses. (We discovered later on that the selfs prefer the scent of mint in order to prepare humans for this kind of contact.) We were also a little anxious because we were not really sure how to give space for the real instructors of the course: the selfs!

Well, we decided to ask Falco. As he often did, he smiled and gave us an answer that instead of resolving our doubts, stimulated even more questions. He said, *"Don't worry. The selfs will let you know when it's time."* Then, he gave us a piece of paper with a few sentences written on it. These were the activation codes for every single exercise. Underneath each spheroself and in any complex Selfic structure, there is a kind of special "keypad" with buttons made of small spheres containing alchemical liquids. These liquids are prepared according to specific, codified procedures that not only consider the material composition of a substance, but also the energetic and temporal ones. Each sphere is associated with certain letters, so by touching them, you can "write" words and phrases.

We were excited and intrigued. It was kind of like a treasure hunt, an "Open Sesame…" magical search for our spiritual treasures. We realized that we were on a journey, seeking clues that could bring about a different kind of understanding. Cicogna and I were the first ones who should have been open to new ways of thinking.

But what exactly does it mean, *"The selfs will let you know?"* What if we couldn't really hear what they said? What if we didn't understand them? How could we conduct this course for two days and an overnight stay?

Back then, Damanhur courses were real immersions into another dimension. We turned off all our cell phones and initiated a journey that began the morning of the first day and ended the evening of the day after. Participants shared all their meals together, often with very unique menus in keeping with the theme of the course. Ours included daring combinations and many surprises in order to stimulate the external senses and begin a process of changing logic… It was interesting, but none of our recipes made it into the official Damanhurian cookbooks!

Nighttime was also part of the program. With the Inner Senses course, we all went to the Temples so we could be in contact with this extraordinary creation and explore new dimensions, even during our sleep.

The first courses were exciting and deep. The selfs spoke "loud and clear"—not only with us but to every participant—and we created a pathway with well-defined stages using both personal and group dynamics. The selfs succeeded in finding a specific communication channel for each person, and at the same time, working with the group, allowing everyone to feel like a cell in a vast and complex being. As we expanded our awareness of the extraordinary nature of each individual, sharing ever more of ourselves with others, we could feel other people's experiences within ourselves. The usual sense of personal boundaries disappeared in a deep and moving communion, while everyone's unique essence shined brightly and became more defined.

"not yet"

We realized that we were encountering intelligences that were different from our own. Falco commented on what we needed to do for this exchange to be meaningful. He said, *"We must have the humility to transform ourselves and not fall into the trap of always remaining how we are, that is, thinking of ourselves in the same way. For each of us, the selves touch on the most useful points, without the preconceptions and constructs that we as human beings have about our species. These 'alien beings' are in contact with various parts of ourselves, and certainly not the most surface level ones, but the fundamental ones within each of us. Perhaps the only problem is that we are accustomed to behaving in a certain way.*

How can we convince ourselves to get out of our mental habits, our perceptive ones too, knowing that they aren't as deep as a sea; they are only rivers, only directions? The fact that we can be convinced of this is an important step, and it is a step that is not understood a little at a time but all at once. The selves amplify the system in order to make it as clear as possible, so we can hear what our minds wouldn't normally let us hear."

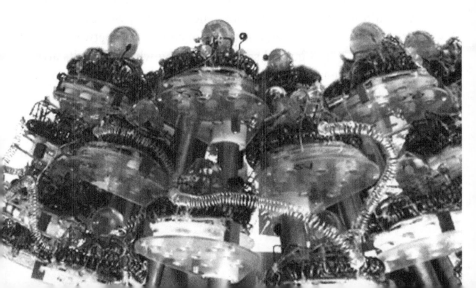

One of the most difficult challenges is being able to accept the extraordinary nature of our sensations, compared to our everyday perceptions. The mind often tries to find an immediate explanation within current patterns of thinking, that is, through the past. Memory interprets what is new by reducing it to something that we already know. We knew that a new way of thinking was necessary, and the selves helped us by explaining the philosophy of "not yet." They said that we humans use absolute negation too often—the "two-letter word," as the selves say to avoid even mentioning it—and this precludes many possibilities. When I am not able to do something or I believe I cannot do it, I should remember to say, especially to myself, that I cannot do it yet, and leave some space within me so that what I desire can really happen—without the anxiety of expectation, simply allowing myself to be present, active and open to the possibility of change.

To make this real for us, the selves guided us in exploratory exercises about states of matter around us that apparently did not exist, ones we could anyhow distinguish by tuning our perceptions into frequencies that were outside the norm, as if we were radios and we could choose which range of frequencies to receive and transform into sound.

Using what we call the "Sense of the Dream" while awake, we could feel and become colors and elements; we could float up into the sky, see the energetic traces of connection between us and everything... in a guided sequence during which the selves always asked us if we could perceive, getting us used to saying "not yet" when the perceptions were not yet well-defined.

We felt that the space of "not yet" brought about a feeling of softness that enabled the heart and mind to work together more easily, to manifest the joyful and creative sides of ourselves. From this place of relaxed and conscious presence, the selves helped us to use a perception that combined what comes from within and moves outward—and as such, having an influence—and not just what comes from the outside and moves inward, as is usually the case.

Staying open to all possibilities, we learned to think with the entire body and not just the head, and we had the feeling that we were undergoing a cellular level "cleansing" process. Touching the divine aspects within us and connecting them to the human ones, it changed everyone's vibration. We could clearly perceive the effect, and it made us feel some very deep emotions.

As Falco often reminded us, *"emotions are a fundamental element, because they can make us feel something with all the different parts of ourselves, all of our personalities, even those who are the most asleep and the furthest away. This is important to fix events in awareness and memory."*

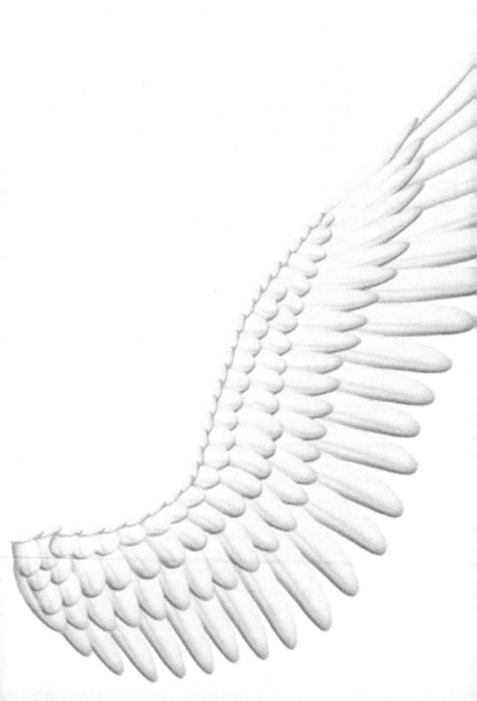

The subtle organs

To stabilize this transformation, the final part of the Inner Senses course was held in the Hall of Mirrors of the Temples, just as it is for the courses that are held today. With the help of the selfs, we have the opportunity to "build" a "subtle organ," i.e. the completion of energetic circuits that transport vital energy within the body. The subtle organ is a new physical and energetic connection that allows us to more effectively use some of our dormant faculties.

Like all profound things in Damanhur, this "activation" includes a bit of humor, to help the mind open to new concepts and dynamics. Over time, we have added different types of organs: tails, wings, spheres, fingers, spirals, mustaches, miniskirts... every form helps us to visualize a different part of the body, to anchor in our cells the energetic structures that we construct with our will, our thoughts and the particular substances that are present in the Temples and "woven" by the selfs.

After all the Damanhurians had experimented with this course, we began to offer it to our friends from around the world. Deborah Malka, an American physician with a doctorate in human genetics, participated in one of those first courses. At the end of the experience, she commented about the experience.

"With the group from the Inner Senses course, I went to the Temples to conclude the course in the Hall of Mirrors. The large spheroself came with us. Cicogna and Esperide guided us in a dynamic meditation with breathing to attune us to ancestral body parts, starting with the tail. I discovered the bioenergetic imprint of my tail! It was made of sapphire blue pearls that trailed from my sacrum to the floor.

I experienced my primal self as an animal with a tail. I sniffed the others around me, and I felt their presence through my skin. Being able to perceive with expanded senses is one of the characte-

ristics developed in Damanhurian seminars, finding lost parts of the self. Only, I didn't know that the activations were for real!"

Today, the "Reawakening the Inner Senses" course is one of the fundamental seminars offered by the Damanhur University. The current version is shorter than the first editions of the course, but participants still have the same depth of experience. For those who choose to be truly present, keeping their hearts and minds open, the selfs guide them on a pathway of expansion that can transform forever their perception of reality.

Paul Taylor is founder and CEO of "Global Citizen", a consulting firm based in Florida; he specializes in strategic media positioning to obtain the greatest positive social impact. He heard about Selfica and Inner Senses for the first time in the summer of 2012, and his discoveries have all the freshness and excitement of our first experiments. Here is a brief excerpt from Paul's relate of his experience.

"After we ended the the first exercise of the inner senses seminar, we went into a period of deep reflection. It was really interesting to acknowledge my need for mental meaning frames before I felt comfortable going into the experience. The Damanhur philosophy suggests that we 'have the experience first, then bring in the mental.' This was difficult for me at first. Part of me yearned to express my experience, but I still felt distant from the group. I found out at the end that this first exercise was about opening, releasing, cleansing, feeling how powerful we are. Learning to deal with frequencies, this art generates constant responses. Speed, geometry, angles, vibrations. The power of saying 'not yet' instead of 'no.'

During the next meditation, I opened my heart and I imagined sending its bright light in a clockwise direction through every person there in the circle with me. I couldn't stop gyrating in fundamental pattern of universe, directing energy through a figure eight infini-

ty symbol, into the divine essence of every soul. Our hearts expanded like stars, and we became one. I fell in love with the Selfica, with the feeling of divine loving intelligence alive in all of us. It is constantly organizing us—more and more cohesion to more and more complexity, so that all matter becomes divine and won't require form anymore. I feel completely resonate with this blissful coherence, which breathes us in and out of existence.

The exercise focused on growing a tail was a very wild experience. The key was to try not to mentalize the type of tail you desired beforehand; just let go and see what emerges. In the total darkness of the Hall of Mirrors, I felt my tail emerge as an extension of my spine and kundalini. It was thick and the sheath began to take form. It was deep turquoise, emerald green, scaly, but smooth to the touch, shiny, and sparkled with light.

Then I heard others in the group sharing their experience. Monkey tail. Panther tail. Dolphin tail. I wanted a dolphin tail too. I never thought of that. Maybe I could will my way to a dolphin tail? No. It didn't work, and it wasn't meant to be. Then I heard someone say that he had a tiger tail, and suddenly a tuft popped out of the end of my tail, and I felt like I had a lion tail. I realized that I must be an emerald green majestic lion. But something didn't feel quite right.

We were invited to start walking around the Hall of Mirrors with our eyes closed to try out walking with our new tails. I immediately felt my hips start to sway back and forth like a lion. Then the strangest thing happened. I realized I had wings: big, powerful wings that extended out of my shoulder blades. I was not just a lion, but a powerful, majestic gryphon.

As I walked around the room, I felt incredibly male in my body, but I also felt incredibly female at the same time. I was wise, all knowing, all seeing, graceful, fierce, powerful, compassionate, regal, and somehow queen-like all at the same time. I was a gryphon, and I was a living embodiment of divine loving intelligence. When we were invited to sit back down in the circle, I chose a seat of power. I was a divine presence in human gryphon form. Many of us had taken our divine stand.

Then on my final night at Damanhur, I took time to walk around the central grounds as if I were a gryphon. I had a deep integration and embodiment experience. First, I hugged the standing stones of the Sacred Ritual Circle; I smelled and tasted the earth in this Stonehenge connected to the four seasons, the Solstices and Equinoxes. Then I walked the spiral of Damjl barefoot, where the idea to walk the grounds in my gryphon form first came through. I activated the circuit energy of the red menhir with my hands and feet, and then I walked through the circuit walks in my gryphon form to help improve memory, use the dream state, overcome insomnia, improve digestion, increase optimism. I fell in love with life and the divine Selfica intelligence again and again and again."

Empowering
the "Microlines"

We also have the "Empowering the Microlines" course now to complete the development of our "refineries" of inner energy, to fully awaken inner senses and get us closer to our divine nature. During this course which offers direct experience, thanks to the selfs, we can more deeply investigate this method of exploring beyond-ordinary dimensions.

With the help of the structures in the Temples, we work with the "microlines," which are the subtle energy lines of the human body that correspond with the energetic matrix of the earth, the Synchronic Lines. The intention is to restore a harmonious and integrated energy system in the body.

We each have a potential that grows in proportion to our chosen objectives, determination, and identification of our life mission. Reorganizing and potentiating the energetic circuits of the microlines is a crucial step for working with our vital energies, because it allows us to create a solid and "clean" container that can support the awakening of *kundalini* in a safe and balanced way.

In our era, much ancient knowledge is becoming easily accessible, but often in a way that is superficial, "adapted" for consumeristic use, or serving a misunderstood idea of personal power. Very often, this involves techniques and practices related to sexual or vital energies that are part of esoteric traditions, which presume a lifetime of dedication with serious discipline and commitment.

Without these energetic and spiritual containers, easy "initiations" and a mix of practices can damage our delicate energetic systems, and instead of creating a deep and lasting pathway toward reawakening, we risk creating a short circuit that makes our integration even more difficult. Using our Selfic "allies" enables us to reinforce and align the human energy systems, facilitating a better integration of mind and body. This creates a solid foundation that can serve as a support for any kind of practice.

Wendy Grace is an artist and philanthropist who lives in California and has much experience in the field of alternative therapies. She shares about her experiences of getting to know Selfica with the Reawakening the Inner Senses and Empowering the Microlines courses.

"These unusual tools have fascinated me since the first time I saw them when I went to Damanhur in 2000. The first one I saw was a mass of copper wire. It didn't look like anything I had ever seen before in the world of art or science. A part of me almost laughed at the apparently chaotic mass of coiled wires, metal, colors, glass and liquid. There are few things in my life that have elicited such a compelling fascination from me.

The first time I came to Damanhur, there was course on Inner Senses being offered, and I immediately signed up for it. I was totally amazed by the end of the seminar. My world had expanded from a world of five senses to a world in which there is a consciousness with sense organs that are vastly more complex, with which I can interact to expand who I am. I, in turn, could share with them my own world and my five physical senses. For me, a Selfic tool was no longer simply a mass of copper coils or an object. Instead, I experienced an instrument that mediated a relationship for me with a living conscious intelligence.

Through Selfica, I was in touch with a new world of beings and possibilities within myself. At the end of my five-day stay, I bought a spheroself, one of the most unusual and costly selfic instruments. I didn't understand it consciously, nor did I have a realistic idea about how to use it. But I had to have it! Why not? I felt like I had acquired some unusual and special friend, and I knew there were secrets to unfold in our relationship. My husband bought me a Selfic painting.

I couldn't have dreamed then of the relationship and the journey that the Selfic beings would bring to me, nor could I have imagined the world of subtle energy they would open to me. Through the activations of the inner senses and the awareness of my microlines

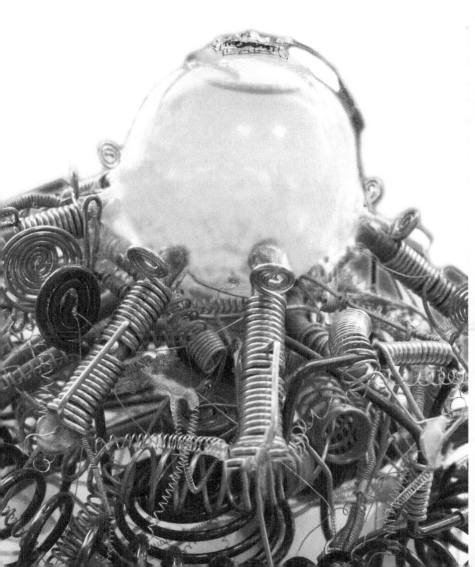

system, Damanhur has allowed me to construct a container which helps my subtle energies to open up, develop, and enter into a larger world. It's as if I have sense organs that can perceive things that I wasn't aware of before.

The Selfic devices have different levels of complexity. The Temples of Humankind in Damanhur are the largest and most complex instrument of this kind on earth. When I was in the halls of the Temples with the Selfic structures activated, I felt a sense of complete wholeness. I felt at ease, as though I were in a familiar place, even if the Temples didn't resemble anything that I had seen before. During the activations for my inner senses, I perceived other lives and parts of myself that I had only intuited before. From there, I began to understand how we are inside a history that is much vaster, a history that is mine and all of humanity's.

With the help of the Selfic instruments, I sense my intuition reaching through time into energies that, when cultivated, can improve the chances for the survival of humanity and its divinity on our planet. I find in myself memories of other worlds, awareness of a much greater river of life of which we are all apart, a much greater purpose and a vastly more complex understanding of life.

Many are awakening now on this planet, responding to the call to return to healthy and sustainable systems. The selfic instruments and the inner senses offer not only great personal growth and expansion, but also very practical applications for this work. Thanks to the dedication of so many at Damanhur, the Selfic energies have revealed themselves and they found me. I am grateful that I can participate with them on my journey into life."

Selfs and senses

During one of the very first courses on inner senses, while the participants were lying down in deep meditation—or better yet, on a "journey" guided by the selfs—I moved close to admire the large Selfic structure that was conducting our work. I thought that the self was just beautiful, glistening in the dim light of the room.

In my mind, I clearly heard someone say, *"You're very beautiful too!"* and I felt a physical sensation, a pleasant shiver that ran through me as if someone had just hugged me... but, from the inside! I stood there feeling completely puzzled. Was this the voice of my vanity looking for reassurance from an alien intelligence?! Then I understood.

Our external senses, those we use to enjoy the richness of the world around us, are very different from those of the selfs. In their form of contact with our space-time—made of metal, crystals, liquids and glass—the selfs cannot walk, touch, taste or smell. However, during the exercises, they can open windows of perception onto our world through us. This sensory ability was the beauty they were referring to.

Cicogna has had many experiences of sensory "exchange" with the selfs, and she told me about one of the most exciting ones. *"During one of the meditations in the inner senses course, I began to feel that my sense of smell—which is already very sensitive—was expanding, until I perceived odors that weren't from the human world! When this wave of sensation hit me, I clearly sensed that it was coming from the self, so I tried to rationalize it and imagine that it was the smell of metal mixed with the glue and crystals. However, I know those scents very well, and my mind knew that this wasn't the real explanation. I breathed deeper and simply decided to let go. I was immediately catapulted into a world made up of pathways of breath, trails of scent, sparking bright connections that were soft and radiant. I understood that the selfs were sending me information about their world, translating through the sense of smell. After the surprise faded, I opened up a space within me to welcome this experience. I knew that reciprocating their gift with my emotions would open new dimensions of contact.*

I better understood that when we learn to perceive what apparently isn't there, with openness in our hearts and minds, we can start to understand how 'miracles' can happen, and this world becomes a place where anything is possible."

Cicogna and I had never understood so deeply before what an extraordinary gift it is to inhabit a human body, with its capacity to enjoy endless sensations that are transformed into emotions, which enrich our lives and help us grow. Feeling the appreciation from these intelligences has changed so much in our relationship with the senses.

Alterations
of space-time

As we were becoming ever more familiar with the selfs, we realized that if we opened possibilities in our minds, the selfs offered us experiences that made those possibilities a reality, or they invited us into new explorations. Cicogna was often "transported" into journeys within the structures.

"I felt 'captured' by the selfs, and I began to move along the copper as if it were a pathway in space. In the Temples, I could see my energetic structure in connection with the Selfic structure of the halls. This still happens to me, and I am always surprised. I understood that we really are more than just our bodies, and the soul is much more than what we can perceive. We are not alone in this space-time, and we share our existence with many other kinds of beings.

Our world is rich with life—or better yet, lives—that are marvelous and complex. In order to have an experience of this, it is important to leave space for constantly discovering something new, rather than bringing everything back to what we already know. Every time I am able to do so, the treasure of knowledge that comes back to me is ever greater.

It's not easy for me to convey these understandings with words, and this helps me to understand the difficulties Falco faced in explaining these things to us. If you don't perceive them directly, you can't know them... that is, as long as our human Sense of Exchange isn't working perfectly. If that were the case, we could fully share the essence of every meaningful experience."

One of the most important episodes that happened to me was when I was in connection with the large self that helped us during the early years of experimentation. I was lying down next to a circle of participants in a course when I heard a voice in my mind, loud and clear, telling me to go to the center. I had already learned not to argue when the selfs give me directions, so I got up and went to the center of the room, standing beside the self. Suddenly, my perception of my body and space had changed. I felt myself transformed into a very tall individual, a man of a different race, and I saw the darkness of space around me. I realized that I was on a spaceship! It was a big, intelligent and living spaceship that I was driving with my thoughts. On his/my left arm, there was an elaborate Selfic bracelet that make my forearm move, drawing signs and codes, as I felt its metallic endings become part of my flesh, very deep within. I saw stars, planets, star bases, and a Temple connected to many worlds.

These perceptions were extraordinary, but what really struck me was that I sensed this man (a future me?) belonged to a People, one in which everyone is telepathically connected and totally aware of being part of a divine force. Thanks to this constant awareness, a perfect symbiosis existed, and even the spaceship was alive and intelligent, because every creature and the entire universe was kept in cohesion by the thought of this divinity. Humans were aware of being a particle of divinity, and they recognized their importance for that Force. This sudden opening gave me a wonderful sensation of a vast and profound order, of being part of a unified whole that is sensitive and intelligent. I began to do research related to memory—of the past as well as the future—which at Damanhur, I have the privilege of sharing with others.

The "Stars"

We have an experience of creating an "energy" spaceship, or "Star" as we like to call it in which we lie down making a circle with all of our heads at the center imagining that every participant is one of the points of the star. This has become one of the classic experiments with Selfica, not only during the Inner Senses seminar, but also as an advanced meditation technique that we now offer all over the world.

Since 1999, I have facilitated hundreds of meditations and "contacts" with the selfs, and I have experienced how easy it can be to move awareness in different spaces, dimensions and consciousness, thanks to the intention of the group and the combination of everyone's essence. The process of creating a single palette with each person's unique color opens the doors of the mind; it brings us closer to perceiving as the multidimensional beings we can become due to our divine nature.

I am always really touched to feel the communion and beauty of what people "distill" from themselves when they create a true union. The presence of the selfic intelligences easily creates a state of deep meditation, even for people who are not used to being still and listening to themselves. When thoughts quiet down, it is easier to feel what unites us rather than what divides us.

The selfs integrate the mental energies of the people present, and they create a "subtle vehicle" that projects a part of consciousness and perceptions into a different space, where the parameters of reality change. We experience a great sense of union with ourselves, with others and with the profoundness of life.

Wendy Grace, a friend from California who has done research in the field of communication and use of Selfica for many years, describes her sensations in this way:

"When I meditate with the Selfic intelligences, I feel a sense of lightness and playfulness in a very deep place within me. When I am lying down with other people for a "contact" using the star pattern, I come out of the meditation with a deep sense of connection with others and with the subtle energies that are beyond my physical perception. I feel hope for life in a new way that gives me strength and centeredness, even in the midst of life's challenges."

Echidna has participated in many explorations guided by the selfs, and because of her sensitivity, she has had lucid and meaningful experiences. *"During all of the contacts with the selfs, I've felt like we were literally taking off. I and the others in the "star" felt as if we were immediately tickled by these presences, refueled with energy and lifted off the ground. The selfs guided us into other spaces, sometimes at amazing speeds, so fast that we could perceive de-pressurization and voids, similar to being in flight. We felt free from the body's limitations; we even felt as if we had super powers, because we let our imaginative thoughts come out, and it had an immediate effect which we could play with virtually, laughing out loud. It was like being a child in an amusement park! Everyone felt the presence of the selfs, regardless of personal differences in the ability to let yourself go. We often described similar images and actions at the same time; we felt the speed and movements of others, the dimensional effects, and the effects of lights, sounds, colors, smells, tastes, emotions...*

These experiments induced expande d states of consciousness for us, an amazing sense of freedom and a deep sense of union amongst all the participants. On other occasions, I've had more personal experiences. I have remembered scenes from different lives and the connections I had with other people in other times. I have reawakened poignant memories from a time in Atlantis, and I have visualized various beings from other species or worlds. Once, I found myself in a drop of water. Another time, I was at the North Pole. I don't know if I was inside or outside of matter. I found myself in front of a huge glacier and became aware that in current times, the glacier still existed due to memory established in the molecular concatenations, and that it wouldn't have existed any more except for the laws of planet Earth. In another contact, I entered into the animal species of my Damanhurian animal name, feeling my instincts and perceiving myself in the body of an echidna. I was underground, using my hard paws to dig into the earth and encountering other beings, prey and company. I sensed presences and information arriving from kilometers away. It was unforgettable!"

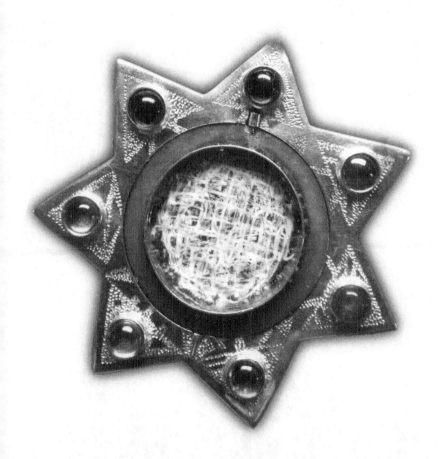

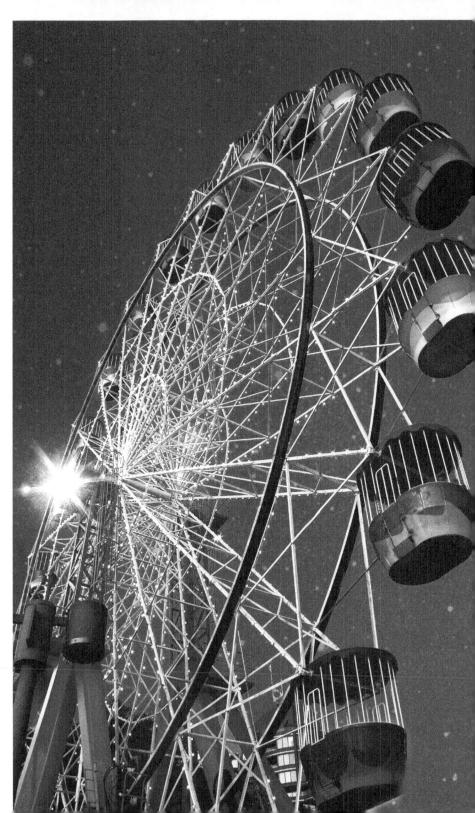

...and the cosmic Amusement Park

In addition to an experience of deep communion with others, experiencing contact with "reality" through the selfs can also be fun. An open mind and a sense of humor are necessary ingredients to transform personal research into a journey full of surprises, as evidenced by David Pearl. David is an opera singer, author and international consultant in the fields of creativity and innovation of organizations. David comes to Damanhur often to relax and find new ideas and inspiration, and ever since his first visit in 1995, he has crossed paths with the Selfic intelligences.

"I first heard the word 'Selfica' many years ago on my first trip to Damanhur, and like many other first-time visitors, I was intrigued by some odd-looking objects in ceramic and glass containing intricate spirals of coiled wires.

Sculptures? Objects d'art? Science fiction souvenirs? No, apparently they were structures constructed to conduit cosmic energy forms.

Err, Really? I was a little dubious, but I couldn't resist buying a couple to refresh the energetic atmosphere in my home and office. When one of them visibly grew like a flower seeking the light, it certainly seemed they were more alive than I had at first believed.

So on my next visit, I purchased a Selfic bangle or two... Okay, I confess, it was vanity. I would have bought them just as pieces of jewelry. The fact that they could apparently help hasten the integration of my personalities or create a shield against harmful radiation seemed to me an added bonus. Bottom line, they looked cool.

I accept that this is the reaction of a fundamentally shallow person, but I am happy to report that Selfica seem a tolerant, nonjudg-

mental bunch and are happy to consort with humans, even when their motives are downright trivial!

My connection with Selfica deepened when Esperide came to London for a workshop and brought along with her what looked like an elaborate hatbox. Nestling inside was not a hat but Esperide's spheroself, a wonderfully intricate sunflower of interlocking coils crowned by a mysteriously fluid-filled bulb. She spoke of—and indeed to—the spheroself as though it were a friend who had flown with her from Italy.

By the way, how did she get it through security at the airport? This was pre 9-11, but paranoia was already rising about terrorism. How did she get this obscure device covered in coiled wires past the vigilant guardians of our Homeland Security? 'Oh, I always tell Customs people it's an artwork,' smiled Esperide, 'and they wave me through.' Esperide is a persuasive person, but even so... I couldn't help thinking that the spheroself must have played its part in this game of ingenious misdirection.

'Played its part? But it's an inanimate object,' nagged the conventional reasoning voice within. That voice used to get particularly strident whenever I visited Damanhur or experienced Damanhurian work.

In the workshop, the spheroself decided to 'put on a show' which left the inner doubter speechless. It seems the Selfica like to play, really play, with humans. They enjoy experiencing our world through our senses, emotions and desires. The spheroself clearly considered the workshop in London a kind of amusement park stocked with playmates.

I remember strong sensations of being abnormally tall, then tiny, then being bounced around on some invisible bouncy castle. At one point, everybody in the room found themselves simultaneously leaning to the right. Then the left. It was like a group dance with an alien partner. It was crazy. It was fun. What else could it be?

Before long, I too was convincing the UK Customs and Excise at Heathrow Airport that my own spheroself was 'an artwork.' Again, no problem.

Then Tricheco, one of the jewelers who creates beautiful selfs in gold and sliver, made me a Selfic ring containing miniaturized circuitry that connects directly to my spheroself in London, so I can now contact her (for a 'she' she is) wherever I happen to be in the world. I do this almost automatically now, whenever I want to open a channel to greater resources, energy or ingenuity. Also, to keep myself and my lovely family safe if we are in challenging situations.

I recently took part in an Inner Senses workshop. After deciding to enroll, it only took about four years to find the time to do it. It's amazing how we let 'urgent things' get in the way of the important things. I can only describe this as a sort of advanced driving instruction for the Selfic traveller. It deepens your connection with your Selfic associates and involves some really cosmic aerobatics. I am still digesting the implications!

The other day, my young son Zachary asked me if he could take one of our domestic Selfica to school to show his friends. I was thinking that kids more normally take a pet along to this sort of show-and-tell, but then..."

Times and places

With some kinds of experiments, it is possible to use the selfs to expand your presence through time or explore the energetic qualities of a particular location. One of the episodes that struck me the most happened at Kathmandu in Nepal. I walked around the Boudhanath stupa until I arrived at the highest point. I had my spheroself with me (this was before liquids were forbidden aboard airplanes, and I always traveled with my beautiful "creature," held in a transparent box covered with stars, which is fitting for its cosmic nature), and I was sitting against the wall of the stupa. It was February, the sun was shining, and I felt a deep sense of peace. I asked my spheroself if it would show me something significant about the place where we were. I breathed deeply and began to do a simple exercise to expand the senses.

Soon, everything changed. First the sounds, then the scents, and after that, I saw a scene very clearly. The land around the stupa was not filled with streets, shops and traffic as it was at the time, but rather it was a huge, barren expanse dotted with small camps that were teeming with life, people and animals,

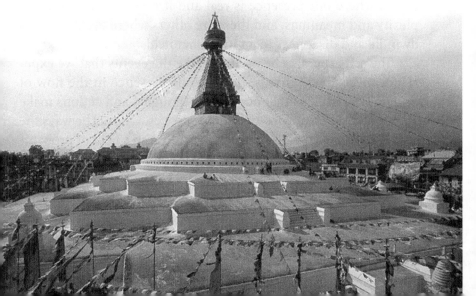

with curtains flapping in the wind. There were many fires lit. The acrid smell of roasted meat drifted through the air and filled my nostrils, mixing with the juniper burning at the entrance of the sloping path leading up to the stupa. I could hear the noises of the camp carried up to me by the wind, mixed with a litany of repeated mantras. I saw a lot of people bringing small, rolled parchments containing prayers and entrusting them to the monk-builders who would then mix them with the earth that they were using to construct a sacred building. I had no idea what era it was, but it was surely an ancient time.

Later, I did some research about the place, and I found out that the stupa was located along an ancient Tibetan trade route. Merchants had camped out there over the course of many centuries, to rest and offer prayers.

When the images faded, I found myself in the usual space-time again, but the surprise perceptions were not over. For a few minutes, I saw an energetic grid that connected all objects. In the inner area of the stupa, this matrix, which I felt was also connected to time, was coherent and orderly, while beyond the enclosing walls, it seemed frayed, more opaque and disorderly. I understood that the density of reality was variable. There are points where our presence is real and it leaves a trace of complexity and meanings, and there are others where events tend to dwindle and disappear in an indistinct field.

The selfs can also be used to make the events that we experience more "real," that is, making our presence in the flow of time meaningful, so that our efforts, thoughts and actions make an impact and create positive consequences. One of the ways the selfs do this is to create an orderly and cohesive field of probability, by literally "tracing" energetic lines of connection.

During a Viaggio in 1998, Sirena Ninfea had an intuition that it would be useful to have mobile selfs, ones that we could take on walks and us, which would leave a trail. With these selfs, we could "write" from one place to another. She proposed this to Falco, who was surprised at first, and then he accepted it as a plausible idea. Then it was his turn to surprise Sirena, because he did not build an object that she could carry around. Instead, he asked her to sit down and take off her shoes, then… he drew Selfic patterns on the soles of her feet!

He used markers that were specially prepared to create Selfic paintings: yellow, green, red and blue ones. It really was a painting, and Sirena's feet were the canvas. From that moment, she would connect all the places she went into the Selfic network, not only by walking there but with every movement she made. Sirena recalls that she went to the Temples regularly because she sensed it as a central point, both as a connection and for "regenerating" the circuits.

Even now, she sometimes feels that when she moves, this memory reawakens and she perceives that the circuits are still working. This wasn't the only time that she has traced while walking. Several years earlier, Sirena walked all over the Car vese area where Damanhur is located, using a Selfic brac "witness"!

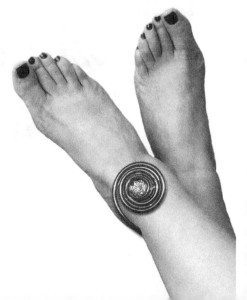

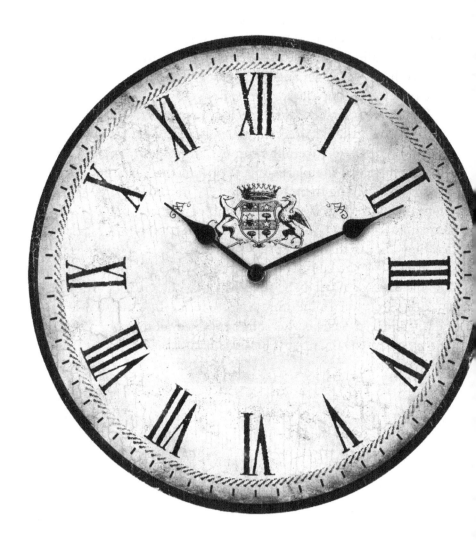

Departures and returns

Human presence and intention are fundamental for activating the "in between space," or the "corridor" between dimensions, that allows the functions of the selfs to meet the field of laws in which we are immersed. They can then create effects beyond the normal cause-and-effect ones to which we are accustomed. "Unusual" effects can manifest themselves because our physical reality is located within a wider dimension: time. Time is a field where events can become manifest, and according to Damanhurian philosophy, it can be interpreted as both a "territory" and a "sphere of the eternal present."

From the first point of view, the space-time continuum that allows the laws of physics to meet up and manifest themselves is not only a container of events; it also puts these events in relationship with one another. Our sensory perception is just one of many possibilities, one that limits us to a single direction—from the past to the future—and as such, to a constant relationship of cause and effect. Events are really connected through the principle of synchronicity. To understand this, we can imagine time as a "sphere of the eternal present" in which all events are simultaneous. Past, present and future are simply different areas that can be put in relation to one another with the right knowledge, rituals and technologies, such as Selfica. The effects seem paranormal only because they do not follow the cause-and-effect relationship that governs our plane of existence.

Sirena told me about a curious example of these abnormalities. *"Many years ago, I had a copper bracelet that I really liked. I felt like it was in tune with me, well suited to my wrist, and I also liked the color it had become. One day, I participated in a 'measurement' competition, or 'metratura' as it is called, a Damanhu-*

rian discipline of concentration. I took off the bracelet to prepare for this exercise, and at the end, I forgot about it. I searched for it everywhere but couldn't find it. I didn't give up, and in my mind, I kept a thread of connection to the bracelet. About five months later, I walked out the front door of my house, which is about 30 kilometers from the place where the competition was held, and the bracelet materialized in the air below my knees and fell onto one of my feet. It was perfect, not only more polished than before, a little more oxidized too. I was so happy! I was a little surprised, but it also made sense that the bracelet finally found me, since I had never let it go."

One of the most interesting aspects of Selfica is this possibility of interacting on the dimension of time. We use selfs for constant experimentation, research in health and wellness, and in magical operations related to exploring possible temporal directions. Sirena personally leads many phases of these rituals/explorations. Her experience shows how interacting with the selfs requires an expansion of normal logic and an understanding that we, as human beings, have the ability to extend way beyond our normal faculties.

"For years, I have been carrying out operations to send out 'time satellites,' that is, structures that can monitor parts of time while orbiting in a space. When I conduct these operations, I become part of a large, open air 'machine' made of tall standing stones, spaces for walking and stone portals to pass through, so that I can use my attention to give the right direction for the 'orbit' of these satellites, which are metal Selfic enclosures containing crystals in stable structures, about as big as a grain of rice. If the operation is done in the right way, the crystals dematerialize in the end, and only the metal shell remains.

Now, I have become an expert and usually everything works well. The first time though, I didn't really know what should have

happened, and the crystal was only scratched instead of demateria-
lizing. I wasn't able to perceive very well the right "time angle" that
I should have found.

This process takes at least an hour, and I feel a connection with
the Selfic structure during the entire time. I continue to follow the
satellite after the launch. Though the portals, I see the path that it
goes on, as if I had another kind of vision. I perceive its velocity, and
I sense the moment when it leaves our dimension.

I sense time as a territory, and the space where I am and time
itself are one and the same. I feel part of a whole structure in an
environment that I can no longer describe… it's dark, soft… Every time I succeed in this operation, I am content and even a little
proud of myself. I am happy to realize that magic exists and that
it is accessible to us, that we can share extraordinary experiences
thanks to Falco's knowledge, which was used to design the whole
structure. Everything is brought about through actions, will, and
the use of thought."

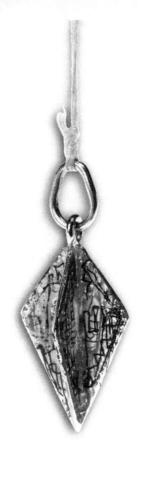

Consultation with the Self

I am always moved when I sense the presence of the selfs, who delicately add something to my normal consciousness. I find it just as interesting and enjoyable to have a "consultation" with the selfs through other Damanhurians who work in this field. In particular, having a look at my health is an important event for me. I consider health to be an integration of the mental-physical and spiritual aspects, as well as the quality of my relationship with myself, with others and the world. I sometimes go to see Antilope Verbena, who for many years now has used a special "Selfic diagnostic board (centralina)" for this purpose. The Selfic part of this sophisticated instrument (Antilope is of course the essential human part of the system) appears as a flat, rectangular wooden box which serves as the base for the use of a gold dousing pendulum.

Originally, it was a table for choosing the right herbal remedy, and it helped identify which treatment to use through a simple binary response, yes or no. Then, its functions were expanded for researching and interpreting the causes for health difficulties and illnesses. Pattens that indicate the main areas of the body were added to the centralina, and the box now has many miniaturized Selfic layers, which are constantly updated as Damanhur's overall "Selfic machine" gradually increases in complexity.

Antilope actives the connection with the person, or in the case of consultations at a distance, with a representation of the person, such as a photograph. Then, she lets the self amplify her sensitivity so she can receive useful elements from the person's energy field, in order to understand the problem. I have used this valuable instrument many times, both for understanding and resolving specific conditions, as well as for expanding my perspective in times of great change.

I am always struck by the depth of the interpretations, the holistic connections with every aspect of life, the centrality of the presence connected to this body, and at the same time, being only one part of a more complex picture that I trace through time, like everyone does. We make a kind of "embroidery on the fabric of time," which allows us to give deeper meaning to every step forward, so that every obstacle becomes an opportunity for growth and ever more true self-knowledge.

Antilope has used this method for many years, and I am not exactly sure where she comes in and where the self intervenes, as it opens doors to other reservoirs of knowledge. She says that it was not easy to open this channel of communication, learning to trust herself and be present, and at the same time, detached enough not to hinder the process: "It wasn't so easy at first. For years I only used the centralina in special places, like in the Temples, going through a process of inner preparation. I felt like I came into contact first with the instrument and then with an ancient and very expert intelligence. I got very tired while doing this, and at the time, I only obtained a few letters and disconnected phrases in response to my questions. I felt a little frustrated, but I didn't give up. Little by little, the answers began to make sense.

I have done over a thousand consultations now, and my channel has grown in terms of quality, strength, sensitivity and emotions. When I activate it, I feel like I am completely lucid, but I am more expansive, and I draw upon other reservoirs of knowledge. If I do consultations about diseases, I always verify the results with the doctors, and my interpretations can be very useful for them in cases where there are different diagnoses.

To begin the process, I ask the centralina if it is possible to investigate something, and I wait for a response. If the pendulum moves to 'yes,' I summarize the issue and ask if we can work on it. If I get another 'yes,' then I say to myself: I'm ready; I focus, and I wait.

I feel the gentle arrival of these forces. I put aside my conscious ego and the energies arrive, sometimes different ones. I always make an audio recording of the consultation, and I notice that my voice changes. Even the cadence of my speech changes to what is most useful for the individual. Sometimes the tone is intimate, sometimes it's more technical, and I'm not the one making the choice. In addition to what I say, I also perceive things, and sometimes I see images that support the words, which I explain right after the channeling.

Elements connected to the person's problem come forth, touching on the deeper implications in order for him or her to really heal, not only to get rid of a symptom. Sometimes the process can lead to memories from other lives, as if the body, in response to a stimulus from this lifetime, were accessing more ancient memories deposited within. I have come to understand that we all carry a story within us, the story of our journey through time, and the body is a stage where many sides of ourselves can manifest, including cellular memories.

The channeling part of the consultation lasts ten to twelve minutes without interruption, and in this time, a lot of things are said! This also changes the energy of the room, and even people who are not used to these kinds of experiences tell me afterward that they felt a great intensity. For me, this work has helped me to better understand the immense powers of healing and transformation that we have as human beings. I feel that I grow, mature, and have flashes of awareness.

I don't think that I have a particular talent, though I have practiced a lot and very methodically, which others have done as well. Selfica has been essential for me to be able to open this mediumship channel which I can use for myself and others. Selfica, to me, has always seemed like something new and very ancient at the same time, as if some part of it were already inside of me. I have always felt fascination and respect when I am face to face with something that is truly alive, not just a simple object.

My relationship with Selfica, with my own Selfic objects and my personal self, is a "technical" emotion. That is, I have created procedures for approaching them and access keys, and when I use or wear them, I really think about activating their functions. My relationship with Selfica has grown over the years, and now that my office is right above the space that houses large selfs used for wellness treatments, I feel like I am in constant contact with them, even in dreams. One time, I felt like I was being called, as if it were a cry for help. I went downstairs right away and found that one of the big crystal Selfic structures had fallen to the ground."

Creating the selfs

Falco introduced the discipline of Selfica in Damanhur, and conducted the most advanced research, but many others have learned to prepare the support structures which host the frequencies of this particular signal and anchor the Selfic intelligences to our dimension. Constructing a Selfic structure is like creating a "body" that is used by the self. In fact, the intelligence of the self is the specific energy that manages the physical part of the structure while continuing to use the laws from its plane of existence to act on ours.

Personally, I have never constructed the selfs. I do not have a lot of manual skills and patience is not one of my strong points either, but I have always been fascinated by the stories of those who create the structures that these intelligences use, because they help me to understand an important nuance of the relationship with these energies. Selfica is not a mechanical discipline, and even the construction of the physical structures requires a precise mind state and a desire to enter into contact with an out-of-the-ordinary dimension.

Over the years, many experiments have been done, and the structures that were first created were not always the most suitable ones for achieving the desired results. In the Selfic studio Selet[12], there is an interesting display case that shows various prototypes and intermediate phases in the development of Selfica, as researchers sought out measurements and proportions that would provide the right key to linking function with form.

12. The Selet studio is located in Vidracco, Italy inside of the Damanhur Crea Center for Art, Wellness and Research.

Some of the prototypes worked, though at times, they displayed eccentric behaviors that left the Damanhurian researchers perplexed. For example, many years ago there was a self for distance pranatherapy which had the vice of extending itself into places where it should not have gone. One of its coils expanded backward, grew and rose up, even if someone wound it back down to the right position every day. This was happening because the structure was defective; the length of its coils was wrong, so the energetic flow tried to adapt the metallic part to itself.

Another funny example of an anomalous one was the Selfica ouija board for automatic writing, which had the defect of levitating at times. Not only did it move around on the table, it also flew around the room. It was pretty complicated for the users to run after it and concentrate on receiving messages at the same time!

Fenice Felce, one of the founders of Damanhur and amongst the first assistants to Falco in the field of Selfica, tells about an episode from the early 1980s in Vercelli, Italy, where he was giving a course with Salamandra on the basic principles of Selfica.

"In addition to theory, the program of the seminar included practical lessons, that is, preparing some kinds of self with copper wire. One evening, the participants of the course were working with various copper wires that needed to be cut with precise measurements, and I was walking around and checking the various measurements to see if everything was going well.

I found an error, a two-millimeter diameter copper wire that was 67 centimeters long instead of 66. I brought attention to it right away and asked the student to cut off the extra centimeter. He said he was being very attentive and was sure that he had measured 66 centimeters, but anyhow, he took the wire cutters, measured one centimeter and cut it off.

Just to be sure, I checked the length of the wire after it had been cut, and it measured 67 centimeters! We look at each other in amazement. I took the wire cutters and cut off one centimeter, and the wire was still 67 centimeters! I didn't give up and cut it again. The wire continued to be 67 centimeters. I was feeling hardheaded and cut a centimeter off the wire and measured it many times over again, and each time, the wire was 67 centimeters. I added up all the one centimeter pieces that had been cut off, and there were at least 20 of them! At this point, I decided that maybe it was best to not keep pushing it. I called Falco and explained what had happened, asking him to tell me what was going on and what to do.

Falco laughed and said that these are the kinds of things that happen when we are involved in a magical science like Selfica, and that anyway, it was best to stop for the evening and try again some other time."

The group of Selfica "builders" is exclusively comprised of Damanhurian citizens, who, just as in the School for Spiritual Healers, have an activation that can progress over time on different levels. It is also necessary to have the right attitude and to be in a harmonious atmosphere in order to construct a self. Cicogna explained to me that, *"If I feel my soul is at peace, I can do the work serenely; otherwise, I run into difficulties. The world of Selfica doesn't want disharmony, and I can't contact them with fixed and schematic thoughts. When I am creating the selfs, I know I must always stay in a dimension of inner transformation. Leaving space within me for the "not yet" is fundamental in our work; otherwise, the parts don't glue together, the coils don't come out right, and I can't continue. Even the everyday things that I have done a thousand times before don't work out."*

Ermellino Ortica, one of the first Selfica builders, and Rondine, who has joined the Selet staff more recently, both emphasize how necessary is to have the right attitude in order to create selfs, because they are not just simple objects. Ermellino shares her experience: *"I began creating Selfic structures in 1986, and to succeed in this work, even after all these years, I must cleanse my thoughts in a way and let go of my worries, because this kind of predisposition makes it easier to tune in with them.*

I learned from Salamandra and Fenice, who were the first Selfica researchers, and I dedicated myself to constructing the selfs with creativity, love and passion, because I have always felt a deep resonance with this world. In those times, there were very few selfs, and over the years, I have identified many other functions which I proposed to Falco, and together we constructed new prototypes.

I also have a relationship with selfs in my dreams. I often dream of structures and constructions made of angles and energies, which I move along as if they were roads. When I wake up, I feel like I've been on a journey to another world that is full of harmony. The greatest gift that working with the selfs has brought to my life is a sense of wellbeing and harmony, a feeling of love that helps me to feel a greater sense of union with myself and the deepest aspects of myself.

I have always had trouble communicating with words; it has been a limitation all my life, but with these intelligences, just like with animals, I feel like I can communicate without having to speak. For me, the Selet studio where I work is a spaceship, a place of arrival and departure for many life forms. Many people come here just to walk around a little, because they say they feel better afterward. I feel really satisfied when I can advise people about the right selfs for them, ones that can bring more wellness and health into their lives."

Rondine: *"From March 2012, I have worked regularly in Selet, and I love it because I can find a familiar energy here, one I can attune with easily. When I walk in the door, it's like entering into a* 'bubble' that harmonizes me and at the same time, transmits many different kinds of stimulus. This is an activity that comes through perceptions and emotions, it facilitates intuitions and inspiration, and it nourishes my imagination. I love working in silence, but because I am also passionate about music, I sometimes select particular kinds of music to play as I am working. Over time, I have noticed that some kinds of music are more in tune with the frequency of the selfs than others, and playing these kinds of music helps me to get in touch with this dimension.

Many times as I am working, I feel like the selfs are guiding me so that my hand movements, the spirals and angles, and as a result, the final products are ever more correct, harmonious and beautiful. When I am at risk of making mistakes, my hands realize it first and send me signals, and only afterward, I move to a more rational level with my mind.

When I began the process of learning how to make the selfs, Cicogna immediately put pliers and copper wires of different thicknesses into my hands for me to experiment with them and refine my manual skills. It's as if my hands needed to activate their memory in order to create the right movements and results.

I feel very satisfied when I see how the selfs bring about joy and positive change in people's lives, sometimes in unexpected ways. For instance, some time ago, a guest came into the shop to buy a bracelet for harmonizing the personalities because she was struck by the positive changes that a friend of hers had gone through after she started wearing the same bracelet a month before. That friend had bought the bracelet just because she liked how it looked! As she wore it, she realized that important changes were happening within her, a transformation that she hadn't expected.

Once, a man who suffered from Tinnitus got the self for hearing. After two weeks, his difficulties were greatly reduced, and after a month, the condition had completely disappeared.

Personally, I have been experimenting with the self for overcoming shyness for some time now. I began experimenting with it a few years ago, then I lost the self. After beginning this second phase of experimentation, I have noticed that I am able to confront the same issue on a deeper level. The self helps me to feel courageous and express things that were difficult for me to say before, finding the right way to do it. It's helping me to speak with others, even sharing personal things about myself because I'm not so afraid about what people might think of me anymore."

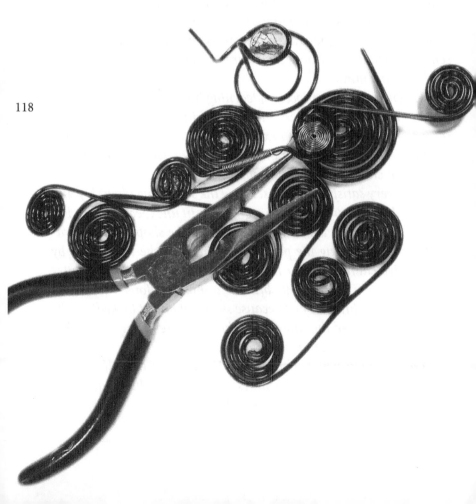

The experience of Cicogna Giunco

The relationship with the energetic dimension of these special intelligences becomes more profound and direct with the passing of time, and Cicogna's story is an interesting example of this.

"*I had my first experience with Selfica in 1983. At the time, I was living in Grosseto, Italy with my husband, and I went to the Damanhur Center of our city. I was pregnant with my first daughter[13], and I had a problem that the doctors wanted to cure with blood transfusions. I was reluctant to undergo this treatment, and so I followed my husband's advice and tried to resolve it through alternative medicine. So, I began going to the Damanhur Center for pranatherapy sessions with Granchia, a healer.*

After a few sessions, the situation hadn't improved, so Granchia proposed that I use a self combined with sessions of breathing in the evening, which are connected to pranatherapy. I was pretty skeptical about the 'magical' approach that Damanhur offered, but when I saw this little, round copper object in front of me, I don't know why but it seemed like it would work. Granchia also gave me a specific graphic pattern to put the self on while using it. I placed the self on the pattern close to me and did ten minutes of deep breathing.

After a few days of this, I began to feel better. I had medical tests done again, and everything went back to normal. I was really amazed by the changes that came about in such a short period of time. After that, I began suffering from headaches, and again I re-

13. Cocorita Camomilla, who is now a lawyer and citizen of Damanhur.

solved the problem with a specific self that I placed on my forehead. At that point, I started to believe that it wasn't just the power of suggestion...

I became an active supporter of the Damanhur Center, and together with eight other people from the group, I founded the Tesan community in Grosseto, which I left in 1985 to move to the main Damanhur community in Piedmont.

Right away, I began collaborating with the Airaudi Studio for pranatherapy in Turin, and I immersed myself in a dimension of healing, helping others and becoming an expert in advising about the most suitable use of Selfica for every condition. In the meantime, research in this field had accelerated, and in addition to the simpler selfs made of copper, there were more complex structures with spheres and many other components. New 'builders' were needed, so in 1990, Falco proposed that I immerse myself in this world in a practical way and learn how to create the selfs. I was happy about this, because I thought that Selfica was the most interesting field in Damanhur and that it would certainly open new doors for me. I came to what I thought was my first lesson full of expectations, convinced that Falco would explain everything to me, and I would have understood all the secrets of Selfica immediately. Something very different happened...

Falco brought out a spheroself, put it on the table in front of me. He smiled and told me to create another one. I was in shock. The structure seemed like an incomprehensible mass of copper wires, wound around in impossible ways! Tapiro, who already collaborated with Falco, gave me a notebook full of notes that seemed even more obscure to me, because his logic of understanding the construction phases wasn't anywhere near mine. Now that I teach how to build selfs, I have understood that each person has a particular way of translating the construction of these structures into sequences and movements.

I only understood the length of the copper wires and the fact that I needed to create coils. I tried to understand the connections between what I later realized were 68 different pieces! I cried a lot, feeling frustrated about not being able to understand, not being good enough and almost reaching the point of admitting my failure. Falco told me not to worry, to take a walk and try again. I felt even more frustrated because it seemed like he wasn't taking me seriously. Anyhow, I went for a walk... which lasted a week, during which I didn't want to get anywhere near a spheroself. Then one day I said to myself, 'Cicogna, today is the day,' and magically, I was able to see how the wires connected up, how they were made, and even Tapiro's notes seemed less obscure.

I succeeded in constructing my first spheroself, and then structures that were more articulated, even arriving at the miniaturized selfs which are my most recent 'conquest.' To prepare myself for their creation, I had 'encounters' with the large selfs that Falco constructed in the last years of his life, which have extremely broad and varied functions. We use them also to connesct to Falco himself, now that he has left his phisical body.

One day, I sat in front of the large self that is jokingly called 'Natalina,' because of the lights that it has which makes it look like a Christmas tree (Natale = Christmas in Italian), and I opened up an inner space of listening. I continued to see ever more intricate patterns, many traces of energy that seemed to project themselves toward me. I understood that they were being deposited into my memory, so that I could recuperate them and use them when it was the right moment.

To create the miniaturized selfs, I also wear a specific Selfic bracelet, and sometimes I feel like my hand is moving by itself, and I just need to stay in the right frame of mind to not create barriers and let what is needed flow. In the beginning, I did a lot of trial runs, and I made mistakes out of fear. Now, I have learned to trust *myself more and it's getting better all the time. My objective is to be able to connect a chosen function with the creation of the structure, that is, to "see" the code of the function translated into metals and liquids.*

I currently teach people who are getting to know this art, in a way that isn't traumatic for them, even if it is difficult for everyone at the beginning. I am also continuing to learn by deconstructing objects that Falco brought to me over time and asked me to study and reproduce. Often these structures have spiraling wires that are so minuscule and tangled that it's even hard to count the number of coils. I can do it though, thanks to experience and intuition, and I often understand the measurements and sequences to follow while in my dreams. Often times, if I make mistakes, indications about what to adjust and modify come to me in dreams.

The relationship with Selfic intelligences involves emotional and symbiotic exchanges. While working to create the selfs, I have realized that this is a real relationship that is established between us humans and the world of the selfs, and it is necessary to learn how to listen. Concentration is extremely important to come into communication with these intelligences, who little by little enter into contact with our dimension.

In the beginning, constructing Selfica is sometimes difficult due to the anxiety of not succeeding, and seeing as how we are rigid, the metal becomes hard too. There needs to be a period in which the tension melts. We need to become soft inside, so the metal softens up too."

Group experiments

After new selfs are created, all of them are experimented with, and the first trial runs are usually done in the context of the Viaggio. Tapiro has a lot of experience in this, and one episode that struck him the most was on the Bovo Marina beach in Sicily, verifying the functionality of a very complex self called the "Arca" or Arc. It was 1983, and at the time, this self had 30 layers of microcircuits, while now it has more than one hundred.

The "Viaggiatori," participants in the Viaggio, present in that moment stood in a circle around the Arc. A transparent glass bottle containing wine was close to the self, because this was the liquid that would test its capacity to act on matter. The duration of the experiment would be determined by some lighted candles nearby. When the candles were consumed, the trial would be over. Tapiro recalls, *"We were on the beach. We had created a circle of presence around the self, and the wine was to become water. We were the motor, the battery, and we provided the human attention in order to interpret the event.*

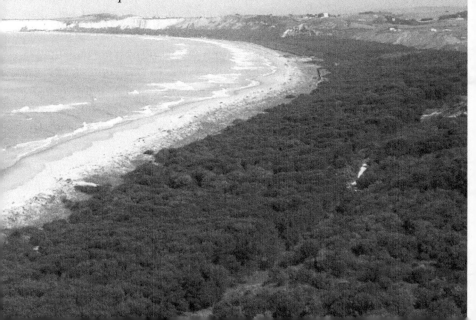

We were the mediums of the experiment. After about an hour, the process had begun, and the wine began to become lighter in color. We were really struck by this, and we participated with ever more intensity. The liquid became more and more transparent until we only saw particles in suspension, which then precipitated without leaving a residue. It had become a bottle of water! We were all very excited, because it's one thing to, for example, see something enter into a box and come out transformed, and it's another to observe the process of metamorphosis with your own eyes.

That evening, we said to Falco that it would have been nice to do the opposite, though he replied that this experiment had already been done two thousand years ago, and it was more complex to transform wine into a completely pure element, instead of the opposite."

Raganella Lilium has been present for the trials conducted in Viaggio for many years now: *"Over time, we have experimented with many selfs, because as soon as Falco finished them, he had us test them to calibrate data and functions. Some kinds of selfs can be programed to carry out various tasks, and they have codes which can activate one program or another. For example, the kind of self that we used to do the first experiences of lucid contact was also used to do work on modifying our memories, an experimentation that gave rise to the 'Transformation of Memories' course, which is now offered at the Damanhur University. In this context, the self had a new activation to act on the branches of time, allowing us to change the interpretation of a negative event from the past, and in this way, transform the consequences that this the event has produced on our way of thinking.*

I am aware that stories like this may seem like they come from a science fiction book. However, by getting into contact with this self, I and those who were present with me had the experience of modifying a specific memory, an episode from our lives that gave rise to some current difficulty. It was a very intense experience. We really relived some episodes of our lives with a lot of emotion, observing them as if they were a film and transforming the final impression of the event into something positive, which consequently modified a current way of thinking. It's as if the self were bringing us to a dimension outside of time where everything is possible, a kind of place-non place where we are able to change mind states and emotions. We saw things from a different angle, and this allowed us to intervene on aspects of ourselves.

One of the first selfs that I remember experimenting with is the 'slittino' or sled. One day, Falco presented us with this strange little self made of silver and gold, which really was made in the form of a sled, and he told us to try it. It was an incredible sensation. Gliding it delicately over the skin, I felt how it was acting deeply on the internal organs, making the energy flow. I felt a great sense of relief in the target areas. In particular I remember feeling a tickling sensation in a part of my shoulder, and I remembered then that some years ago, I had problems precisely in that area.

I also remember the trial run with the large sphere, which is now part of the Selfic system in the pranoself studio. The sphere is comprised of many layers of copper circuits that weave together in a network. Looking through this sphere makes you see reality in a different way. We tried looking at a landscape and then looking at it again 'through' the self. I felt as if I were seeing with someone else's eyes, which was a very interesting and emotionally moving sensation.

The Selfic cube is also an interesting 'creature.' We experienced that it is connected to the temporal and emotional flow of people. It is a complex structure which, in addition to spirals and cages of copper, contains small bottles of liquid in which the Viagggiatori have 'deposited' emotions and feelings from different periods of their lives. You feel this distinctly when contacting the self.

125

Even if you don't know about it, you find that you perceive yourself as if you are in several temporal points contemporaneously, experiencing many different emotions in the same moment.

Since the summer of 2013, this selfic cube has been used by dozens of Damanhurians investigators in connection with the new technology of "Dimensional Portals", that Falco developed until the time of his death.

It's not so easy to translate perceived sensations into words, and it's always a new and interesting experience, mainly because of this way of experimenting in groups. Comparing my results with others, I realize that the sensations I feel always have so many similarities with those of others, even if they are translated into different examples. This assures us that it is not only the result of the mind, but something 'real' that happens."

Selfica and Health

Selfica in relation to health is one of the main research fields in Damanhur. It is a vast and fascinating subject which could be a whole exploration in and of itself. So because of this, I will only mention a few brief points here.

Like other Damanhurian spiritual healers and many other healers worldwide, I use Selfic instruments to support well-being and harmony, with excellent results. The tool I love the most is what we call the "stiloself." I like it because it is so versatile and can used for self-healing too. It is a small wand composed of a body in gold and a head with Selfic microcircuits.

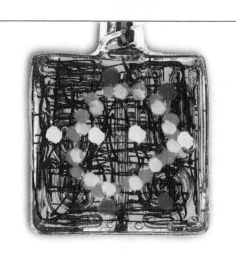

Many years ago, together with a group of Damanhurians who had already used the first spheroself prototypes, I participated in some research sessions to test the performance of the stiloself and give Falco useful feedback in order to expand on it and make it even more effective. We verified that the stiloself works at different depths in the organs and systems of the human body—as well as those of animals, who respond very well to these treatments—depending on how the stiloself is held and if it is put directly in contact with the skin or not.

As with all instruments that create a contact with advanced Selfic intelligences, the stiloself develops a relationship in communication with the therapist who uses it, often "guiding his or her hand" and amplifying empathic faculties so that the treatment is as effective as possible.

Orango tells about how the immediacy of this connection and guidance from the stiloself took him by surprise: "*My first encounter with a stiloself was overwhelming and difficult for me to integrate, because I really felt that there were forces that were more complex than me who were guiding the movement. While doing treatments with people, I intended to run the stiloself along a pathway*

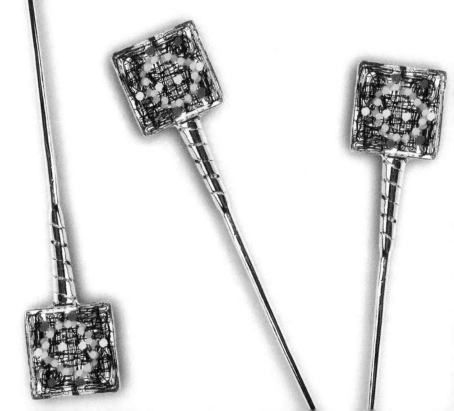

of the body that I had in mind based on experience and knowledge, but the stiloself often influenced me go along a different one. I had to find a balance. At first it was embarrassing. Then when I relaxed, it became another stimulus that I could learn from."

The stiloself conveys the necessary information for restoring balance to organs and systems that need attention, activating the natural intelligence of the body and allowing it to reprogram itself so that it regains its normal way of functioning.

Every stiloself is able to "learn" and increase its effectiveness with each use. Also, because it is connected to a spheroself that supports its complexity, each stiloself is networked with every other stiloself in use on the planet. With these connections, it can tap into information about conditions that it has not treated directly, but which have been addressed by other Selfic instruments.

Deborah Malka, an American doctor who spent several months in Damanhur, was present during our first experiments with the stiloself. She shared her experiences with the Damanhurian doctors and healers, and afterward, Deborah compiled her experiences in writing. In one of the passages dedicated to using the stiloself, she describes how her knowledge of this instrument's potential has grown over time.

"Groups of healers who used stiloself in their treatments were holding some meetings together. This is a typical aspect of research at Damanhur: small groups get together and ask each other questions to discover answers and learn from one another. I attended a few meetings to discover additional uses for the stiloself. I presented my experiences in using the Selfic wand to balance the aura, activate the microlines which are the energy lines of the human body, activate the acupuncture points, and to act as a dowsing tool.

The most unusual thing about working with the wand is that it is like using a tool with a mind of its own. It often pulls my hand along an electromagnetic field that I otherwise would not have been able to feel. I learn from it and it learns from me.

The understanding about Selfic devices is that they can all interconnect to form a 'group mind,' so they share information and experiences. As I share with my wand, I believe it has been my doorway into the Selfic world, and I have been its doorway into my world. It's a real alliance.

My first real encounter with what I call my 'stiloself ally' happened about one year after I'd been working with the wand in my medical office in California. I had already realized that my wand was not an inanimate object, and that the knowledge and impetus transmitted through it did not come from the same pool that I could access without it. When accessing intelligence outside my normal scope, I realize there are so many realities and that being able to organize a greater structure of the 'all there is,' is really only a means to overcome the limitations of my belief systems. Damanhur is in many ways such a catalyst for this process.

There are infinite technologies, but allowing the possibility of just one new pathway to expand the envelope of my psycho-intuitive-rational-body-mind, has brought me one step closer to expressing more of who I am. So the questions are no longer black and white. Alive or not alive, but rather how to best interact with the vast, creative knowledge to which I am having ever greater access.

My stiloself is a tool that is also, in moments of three-dimensional time, evolving, transducing new information and acting alive. There are many forms of life. The beauty of Selfica is the opportunity to experience a different configuration of life that is non-organic, yet still we can communicate.

When I met its being, it really touched my emotions, as if I'd made a friend. I was treating a woman with her left kidney removed many years previously due to a tumor. I wanted to revitalize the left side of her body with the yang force of the kidney meridian, and the energetic subtle-force of the kidney organ, both of which were clearly deficient and had been for many years. I held the stiloself above her body. I thought I would use it to transfer the imprint of these energies from the active right side to the curiously vacant left side. Within seconds my body started to produce huge rivulets of sweat, rolling in beads down the front of my chest. The wand seemed to vibrate with a power surge that sent tingles up my arm and into my chest.

There was a naturopath with me in the room who had treated this patient for many years. I asked her to hold the stiloself for a few moments while I divested myself of the charge. She and the patient both had unusual capacities, ones that I do not carry: they can see the subtle energy of beings.

They both looked at a point behind me and said, 'Oh, there it is, the entity of the stiloself!' The client described it as a gossamer, a subtle-shape. The healer sensed the love and the goodwill of a fellow healer. I couldn't see a thing, but sensed an androgynous presence, both male and female. Do they have healers in the Selfic community as we do? It seems so.

I felt my emotional body respond as I never yet had while working with the stiloself, as if I was meeting a friend. I greeted it and made a pact to be allies in healing. I asked it how to use it without getting blown out, without taking on too much energy for my circuits. After all, I have been doing energy balancing for 25 years and learned long ago how to keep the energy of my client separate from myself, and I had never been overwhelmed with electromagnetic tingles before.

The answer has been a special gift between healer allies. The stiloself said, 'Let the energy flow through the sacred geometric life force fields of your system and all the necessary transductions will naturally happen.'

The transduction of energies from dimensional fields that I had previously not carried in my capacity as a conduit for others couldn't *be held by meridians or chakras, or breath alone, the carriers I had previously used. Now, at last, I would have the opportunity to learn of these sacred geometric fields from a direct experience of their amplification through the force of the wand. Then I asked Falco if he could indicate the patterns and functioning of these fields, and he gave some lessons on the subject.*

Even now, the stiloself still teaches me so much in a concrete way. I have learned during many years of working with the wand that it does not come alive in the same resonance in every case when I use it. As always in healing, the client's state of readiness is integral to the process. At times the effects are subtle and not perceived at all. At times they are monumental and are marked by great changes in the client and in myself."

The stiloself's effectiveness can be accentuated by using the Selfic "slittino" or sled, the silver instrument with microcircuits that Raganella described. It is the one that traces surface energetic lines, which become points of preferential flow for the information conveyed by the stiloself.

The stiloself and the slittino are some of the most well-known and widespread "portable" selfs. In Damanhur, we have successfully experimented with many other kinds of selfs, from ones that are used a few times a week in cases of acute conditions, to very large structures for cellular rejuvenation that are used one to four times a year, depending on the needs of the individual.

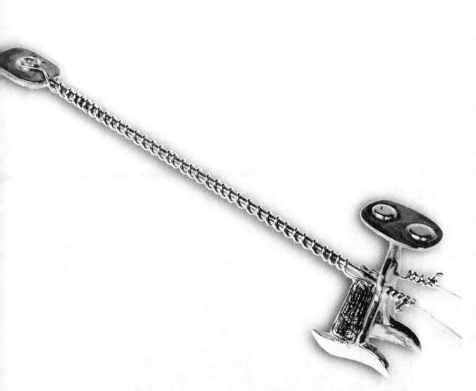

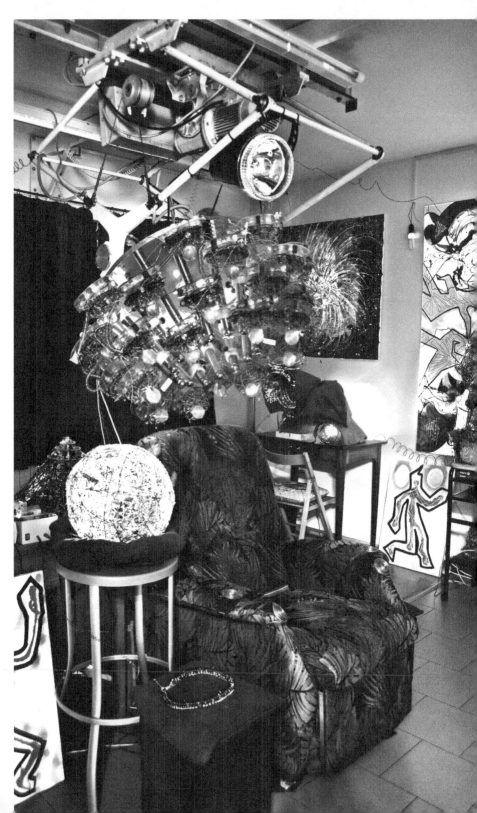

"Pranoselfic" healing

The Damanhurian School for Spiritual Healers teaches that when healing the physical body, a person's past is healed, and the effects that past decisions and events have produced on the present. On the other hand, when we intervene to help a person's aura "shine," strengthening the immune system and the body's capacity for self-protection, we heal his or her future, because on our energetic level, events arrive in a potential form before they manifest on the physical plane.

When we take energetic healing and add the specialized intervention of the selfs, which have an effect on synchronicity and can therefore modify our relationship with time in a positive way, the effects that occur can be very rapid and profound.

You can experience the latest applications in the field of Selfica, connected to the use of energies for healing and wellness, in the "Pranoself" studio at Damanhur where specialized healers operate.

Because of the Selfic structures present in the studio, the "drop" of prana that the healer adds to the person's life force, which acts as a catalyst, is amplified many times compared to a normal session of pranatherapy. This prana returns to the client, who can use the mind to direct the energy where it feels most needed.

In addition to helping me to stay healthy, when I go into the Pranoself studio, I feel like I am getting aboard a spaceship. When I sit in the chair for the session, I seem to be at the command post, ready to receive orders for take-off and explore another part of our wonderful universe.

Section two

SELFIC
PAINTING

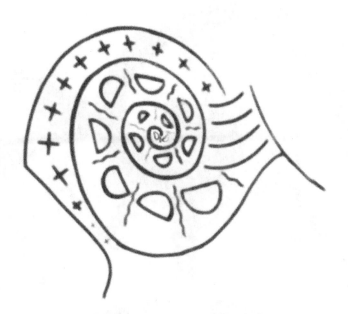

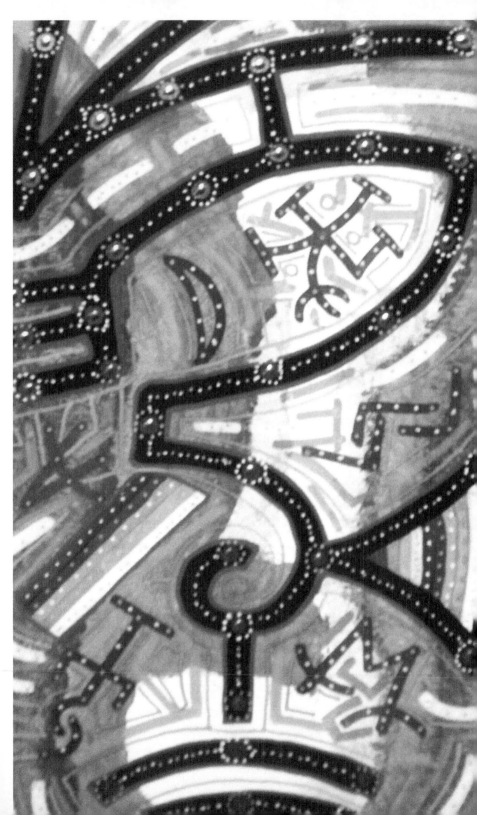

Selfic Paintings

If building an emotional and cognitive relationship with intelligences conveyed by structures made of metal and inks might seem a little strange—if only because you need to accept that this is possible—it is a lot simpler to have an experience that touches the soul through encountering a work of art. So at the beginning of the 1980s, Falco created "Selfic Painting" which adds an aesthetic dimension to the functionality of Selfica. In this way, emotion is the catalyst for a connection with the energetic aspect of Selfica.

Falco's painting is strong, joyful and expansive. It is a celebration, a constant expansion of awareness, a love affair with life and its origins. Falco offers a journey of continuously discovering new forms; his first paintings present harmonious and rigorous relations of lines defining a space that seems to contain, in a compressed form, the vital tension of the universe itself.

Then came the canvases in which the universe itself is the subject, and later on those dedicated to themes-symbols such as keys, cups, the Tarot, chimeras, hands, books, trees. In every instance, the paintings are asymmetrical, sustained and made dynamic by a delicate equilibrium of multi-layered imbalances, different vanishing points, rhythmical yet never repetitive geometries. Sometimes the painting expands onto its frame filling also the space around it with its exuberant strength.

So, many people have developed a relationship with the special energies of the Selfic paintings, which offer profound experiences and emotions. For me, these emotions most of all translate into "love" and "memory." Like many other people, I feel that even though the Selfic paintings may seem like objects, the primary ingredient in these works is life, life as emotions, communication, asymmetry and movement.

In Selfic paintings, the pulsation of the creative act is always present, as if a particle of time had crystalized on the canvas. The painting is there, finished, but it is as if it were still being painted, as if the forms and the signs were continually recreating themselves.

Nietzsche said, "*I have never trusted an idea that came to me while I was sitting still and thinking*," and Kant used to walk under the moon to move his body and way of thinking. Behind Falco's paintings, it is difficult to imagine a static painter. The colors, symbols and forms are the living actors of the composition. Because of this, Selfic paintings seem to have the power to give those who look at them a little bit of extra energy, a flash of new understanding about realty and about themselves.

The permanent exhibition of Selfic paintings in the Niatel Art Gallery of the DamanhurCrea center in Vidracco, Italy is open to the public every day of the year. On display are many works created from 1985 to 2013. Their interaction with each other creates a special space for meditation, which is always available for everyone.

Falco left his physical body on June 23, 2013. His paintings represent a very important part of his spiritual heritage. To continue writing this great Book of Knowledge, before dying Falco trained three Damanhurian women and one man to become his channels and create selfic paintings. Their works have his energetic signature and connect to the same reservoir of energies. The experimentation and exchange with these special intelligences can so carry on, and new doors of exploration continue to open.

Find the one
who chooses you...

Very often, people who have just arrived in Damanhur and do not really know anything about Selfica feel attracted to a painting, almost as if they were "called" by it, so much so that they want to buy it. They do not really know why, but they feel better when standing in front of that canvas. It often surprises them to read the subject of the painting in the title, because it refers to something that is close to their hearts, something they are going through in the moment, or it offers a suggestion or an answer. Over the years, many people from all over the world have become admirers and sometimes collectors of Selfic paintings.

David Pearl tells about his first experience acquiring a Selfic painting. *"They had told me, 'Wander round, take a look, and see which one chooses you...' No, I wasn't in the market for a puppy or pet rabbit, but in the gallery of Selfic paintings at Damanhur, looking to buy my first Selfic painting. As it turned out, the advice that I was given was absolutely appropriate, just like the pet shop analogy. After all, they weren't objects, more like 'living beings,' and they all seemed to be looking at me with puppy dog eyes, saying 'take me back to England with you!' As I wandered around the gallery, the paintings loomed out of the darkness and UV light. I waited to see which one would irrevocably choose me (not the other way around). It was a vivacious swirl of red, pink and gold. When I flipped around the painting I had chosen to discover Falco's description of its use, essentially to stimulate creativity, it couldn't have been more appropriate or helpful for my office, where it still hangs."*

Falco used colors that are visible in diverse light frequencies, so there are different images, compositions and meanings that share space on a single canvas, depending on the color of light that is illuminating it. In this way, every painting is many paintings because different lights reveal layers of symbols and unexpected depths. Every painting can be observed in natural, colored and ultraviolet light, as well as in the absence of light, and in each circumstance it will show a different composition offering a different meaning.

The variations of light that reveal different paintings on the same canvas also recall the natural rhythms of day and night, as well as the flow of time, which is often a protagonist in these works, in a weaving of the past, the future and the eternal "now." This is a circular time in which the stellar origins of humankind anchor themselves in the now of our earthly experience.

Every painting is a doorway, and the path that opens is different for each person who observes it: it is a dream dimension with new laws, an Alice in Wonderland world where everything is possible. Logic is turned upside-down, multi-faceted, non-linear and surprising, always led by the emotions that come about from exploring what is within us. In this way, every painting is a mirror, and Falco often used mirrors in the paintings, creating a play of reflections and gazes in which the painting and the observer study each other reciprocally. The symbols and brushstrokes of the painting take on different forms and meanings, almost as if they were blots from a spiritual Rorschach test, in which everyone can see a reflection of themselves and their own inner worlds.

Crotalo Sesamo's story is a good example of this. Crotalo is a facilitator at the Damanhur University and an Ambassador of Damanhur. "*My first experience with the Selfic paintings was also the most striking one for me because it coincided with my first visit to Damanhur. It was October of 1988, and I was eighteen years old. I was a tennis instructor, and I had felt a spiritual calling for some time. I was fascinated by the mysteries, and Turin, my city,* was the ideal place for this because it has a long esoteric and magical tradition. This interest of mine was the thread that brought me to Damanhur. A photographer friend of mine was working on a piece about the magical places of Turin, and he asked me to identify the most interesting ones. He gave me two books to read. The first one was called, Turin, Magical City, written by the researcher Giuditta Dembeck, who had dedicated a chapter to Damanhur and one to Oberto Airaudi. The other one was a book on the spiritual healers of Damanhur. I read the first one and put the second one on my desk, where it stayed for several weeks. Till the day in which I perceived a kind of luminous aura around it...

This phenomenon really struck me, and I read the whole book in one sitting. After a few weeks, I decided to visit Damanhur with a friend of mine. We were the first ones to arrive and the last ones to leave that evening.

It was a Sunday afternoon, the only time that the community—which at the time had less than a hundred residents—was open to visitors. The Temples were secret and the only thing you could visit was the first settlement, which is now called Damjl. I discovered that the Damanhurians were involved in all the things that interested me, astral travel, dreaming, paranormal faculties and natural medicine... I was feeling enthusiastic, and the biggest surprise was yet to come.

I entered a room with a low ceiling where different colored lights illuminated three of Falco's large paintings. The one in the middle immediately attracted me. I sat down in front of the canvas and... I literally sat there stunned for more than two hours! I didn't know anything about Selfic energies, but I felt as if I had been projected into another space, another time, maybe a place in the future where I had originated from in some way. I didn't understand anything, and at the same time, I understood everything. I had become extremely small, and I felt like I was walking along the lines traced on the canvas, which continually changed depending on the color of the light. Even if my body was still and I sat motionless in front of the painting, I was dancing above the symbols in a labyrinth where I continually lost and found myself.

I was in a lucid trance accompanied by a strong sensation of joy and pleasure. It was a calling of the soul, like a signal for me in the ocean of time... The painting was one of Reawakening, to help me remember, and it seemed to be singing a magical formula, a song. It was like a mantra that revealed my soul to itself and explained why I found myself there, why I had set this appointment in time with myself. It also showed me parts of my future.

When I later discovered that the painting was dedicated to an ancient epic writing called "The Poem of Anansal," my emotions went even deeper. It became clear to me that I wanted to live in Damanhur, and soon I moved to the community.

The painting was owned by a couple, and I was certain that one day it would be mine. So, first of all, I convinced the owners to leave it in a public place so that everyone could see it. The painting was so moved to the welcome area for guests, which I passed by every day to go to the space that in the meantime had become my office! Then, after eight years of asking, I received the opportunity to acquire the painting in 2006. Now, the painting is in the Niatel Gallery, available for everyone to see. You never know, someone might have the same experience with it that I had!

I have become a passionate collector of Selfic paintings, and I have ones from every historical period and every series, from the very first paintings of the 1980s to the most recent ones. For me, these works are like a complex kaleidoscope through which I can see and feel different facets of myself and my soul. The first hook in selecting a painting is always emotional; I always pick them from my gut feeling, because I sense they connect to my emotions through my belly. Selfic paintings give me this sensation of being at home. When

I am with them, I feel like I am projected into a world where I feel more complete and real.

Over time, I have realized that the paintings that I chose—or that chose me?—have some characteristics in common, as if they all bring into focus the parts of myself that I wanted to develop or transform.

In many years of teaching, I have shared my love for seeking knowledge through Selfic paintings with many people. I try to convey a journey of unveiling the most profound parts of ourselves. The archetypal symbols of the paintings serve as access keys for the codes of the soul, which allow us to find parts of ourselves that haven't been revealed yet. To find your own painting, you need to do more than just observe it; you need to feel it and discover if it calls out to a part of yourself, because it is a fractal of your soul.

Lastly, I also use the paintings to train my subtle perceptions, specifically for astral travel, which I have been practicing and teaching for many years. Sometimes during my experiences outside of the body, I have the sensation of traveling through the lines of the paintings, which allow me to enter into different lines of the Beyond, ones I otherwise wouldn't have been able to access."

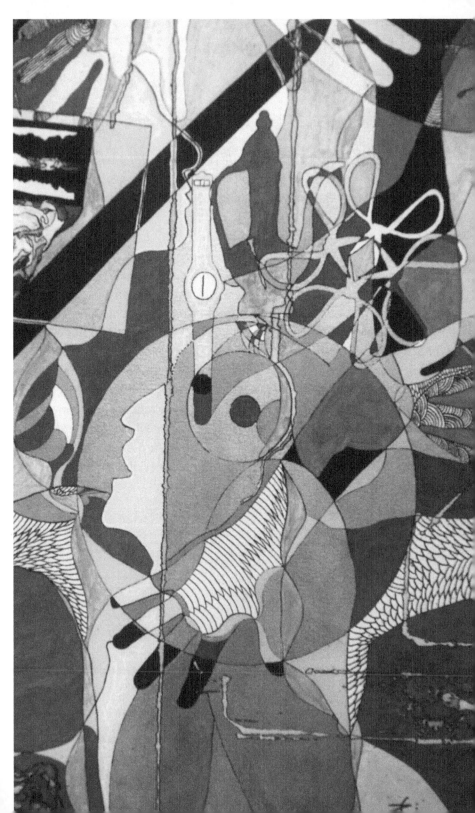

Not paintings but books...

Every Selfic painting is a page from a book of knowledge written with alchemically prepared colors and components, combined with forms and signs passed down from ancient mystical and esoteric traditions. For this reason, Falco preferred to define himself as a writer rather than a painter. *"More than a painter, I consider myself a person who extracts pages from the diary of time, pages on which my experiences are told: experiences of subsequent lives, of knowledge, of my story throughout the millennia.*

All the paintings that I have been painting over the years are the same painting considered from different positions and approaches that represent a complete ecosystem. They are all pages that speak, offering explanations of the same thing on different levels and, as it happens in magic, the story becomes substance, so these pages can, in turn, project all that they contain to their owners, to observers, to those who interact with them. The objective of any research related to these kinds of spiritual aspects is the development of knowledge and of the energy within oneself."

Sometimes, the paintings even indicate which "Book" they originate from. An example is a series from 1996 whose titles give precise instructions:

From the Book of the First Dream:
a whiff, emitted by the divine power
inspirational, ally to those who seek the light
inside their red heart...
So those who lead their steps along the paths of life,
can count on the long pole that finds in the grass
the hidden danger...
So divine breath moves things
to speak with humans...

From the Book of Knowledge:
a solid objective, an inalienable principle,
an ideal, is to be respected for life,
also in the time of reduction;
in this way you are worthy of nobility,
beyond the limits of those who are below the human limit...
Pure power respects the whole,
the decision in alignment with the yearned for knowledge,
for application to Will...
I help to support weak limits,
making them taller and able to overcome the flood...

From the Book of Distances:
a spell leads to goals,
and distance, illusory, makes the steps weaker,
only due to the impression given
by the days needed for the return...
But the wise ones bring all of themselves
with themselves,
like the snail its home...
We are all where the energy directed
on the appropriate directions wants...

Words of Power from the Temporal Book,
coded into measures to the times which are variable
in thickness and substance...
so the temporal weight of an action can be assessed,
its direction and relative measurement
when requesting the evaluation...
I help find ways to better use one's personal time,
in the actions related to work, and for oneself...

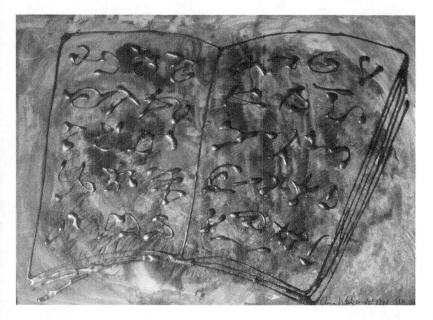

The need to hand down this great book of knowledge, this "history through the millennia," is one of the things that spurred Falco to be so prolific, as he has painted thousands of paintings. The works of Falco offer a taste of "other" worlds, and they suggest infinite possibilities of expansion for the human heart, mind and spirit. His canvases urge us to ask ourselves: what is humanity's place in the universe, and how many realities we could participate in, and which ones, were we only more aware.

Observing the works exhibited in the Niatel Gallery also allows us to understand Damanhur's historical, social and spiritual development, as Falco always stimulated and poetically indicated avenues for Damanhur's growth through his paintings.

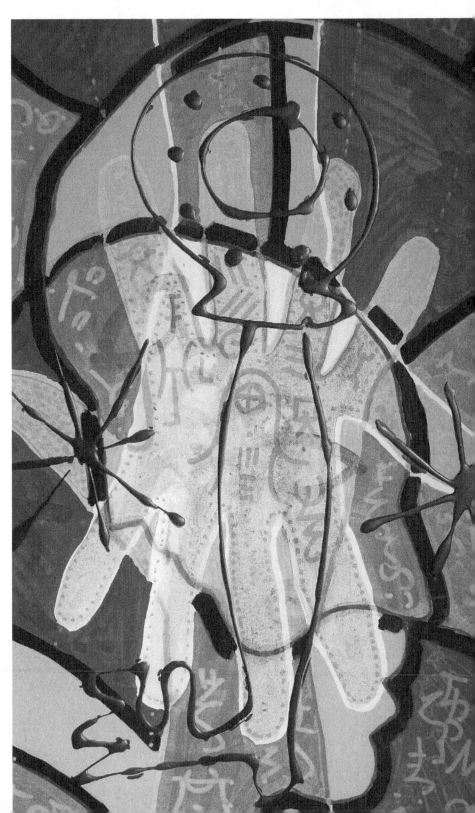

Titles and keys

The titles of Selfic paintings are expressed in a poetic form, and Falco often wrote them on the back of the canvas. This combination of the text and the painting provides the key for interpreting the work. The title expands on and develops the pictorial message, suggesting codes of interpretation and combining the poetry of the word with that of the image, in order to offer a more complete and profound emotion.

The paintings are musical, not only in the harmony of the composition, but also in the interweaving of the sounds of the words, which when read, travel through space and expand the painting's field of existence.

The ensemble, the whole,
the manifest as well as the unmanifested,
create bonds that the wise person, the alchemist discovers...
everything is hidden, everything revealed.
Veiled again, that is, once discovered...
Here is the test to overcome,
the trial that turns students into teachers,
thus perpetuating the teaching.
The beyond, the when and where are children to free will...
choosing what is true and therefore not illusory,
at least once per lifetime,
without then going back...
and reveal/re-veil so that others can discover...
or we ourselves,
in another when.
1988

Being able to combine parts of oneself, to distinguish,
choosing also things that are difficult,
makes you free...
In this way life selects the winners,
while those who accept passively
and justify themselves,
live lives halved of meaning.
What are the things that really matter?
Existence creates things and ideas,
new opportunities of time,
not only reproduction to give physical life...
Daring, leaving a sign, being a human people.
Riding existence...
2008

The titles, written in free canon, intertwine with the sensitivity of those who read them, as indicated by Falco: "*Selfic paintings combine basic forms, colors, ancestral symbols and other elements that are linked by a series of key phrases corresponding with the title. A Selfic painting is a book, and it is important to learn how to read it by observing it, taking in the effect that it produces as a whole, as it moves through and penetrates the senses.*"

Table of Power, with the ancient primary words
and the voice of leading, of guiding, of memory...
He who walks on the narrow roads of the world,
has the opportunity to expand the path,
and make sure that every way will lead to joy,
to the peace that the united soul builds...
With the word of the powerful book, languages are one only,
and gestures can be interpreted in one way only...
1996

"The title is there to generate a state of mind and spark an emotion which may be guided in order to access various levels within the painting. It often includes an ellipsis so the owner can add to the text whatever they feel is appropriate."

Turn on your heart,
give space and way to the sky...
a fluid movement that opens mind,
sensations, games that lead beyond...
1999

Mirror for serpentine dreams,
for those who dare to overcome
apparent limits and impositions,
and explore new ideas and aspirations,
those who later enrich the existing incarnation...
not without courage,
not without intellectual effort,
but this is possible and exciting...
1996

The emotional heart of things:
the value of feeling, of profound being,
not appearance.
Complete Love, who does not ask,
which gives without thinking
of getting something in return...
Divine Love of the highest level,
which is also in you.
If you fear, you lose.
If you give, you gain the absolute...
2001

The split mirror of your heart
reflects intermittent love:
you dare not say, you hold on,
but do not be afraid of change...
2009

"*Often when you finish reading the title, you are almost invited to start again. If you pay attention, the second reading will open new interpretations to what you just read. This can happen over and over again, as if it were a mantra of knowledge rather than a mantra of repetition.*"

Will you remember me?
I am painted inside of you.
The sign you see is a tuning fork
that opens, if you so want,
the room.
1986

Schemes and circuits of the mind,
open to the owner new, unexplored
paths of the soul ...
2011

"*So, the title is a door, a passage that gives the viewer a way to determine how to enter into relationship with the painting. By opening these pathways, it is possible to extract knowledge from oneself that is already present but usually difficult to read. In this way, the paintings become instruments to connect aspects of your own thought.*"

30/10 PORTO 1986

Cimbali; conchiglie; braccia; tamburi;
battono le mani; canti; scalpitio muggiti
e belati; pianti; risa di piccoli; e di
adulti; paura, avventura, senso della
scomparsa, eccitazione, fremito, coraggio,
preghiera, vibrazioni basse e profonde,
tremano i vetri; e le colonne, un peso
avanti; la coda, aspetto, un altro
peso, e cantare sieno sempre nero,
passano e spariscono, tira il vitello altro
di soglia come faremo a rivederci i conigli;
e non sono addormentati; self, niente
altro metallo; suono, tocca e va, taccio; la
bocca ora ho piena di sensi; trattengo
il respiro, salto ...

DIMENSIONALE

I open roads in the mind,
memories and distant recollections,
making them accessible and useful in the now...
I enrich the latest feeling...
2005

Flower of hope
vital synchronic concentrator of opportunities,
bringer of new energies...
2006

I gather and modify your image:
I complete, in a discreet way,
what is missing, I take away and add,
I paint you seen from the profound, in the essence...
2008

Scheme of amplification of the self
to touch unexplored parts of one's mind,
reaching and defining secrets
from other lives and experiences...
Guide to the center...
2011

A painting style that can't stand being rushed...

Eraldo Tempia Valenta is an expert of modern art, and he owns one of the finest collections in Piedmont, Italy. A longtime friend of Falco's, he is called Parsifal by Damanhurians. In the introduction to the book Selfic Paintings, published by Val Ra Damanhur in 2004, Parsifal writes about the connection between each painting and its title.

"Falco painted thousands of paintings and never explained their meaning, but he always accompanied each painting with a 'narrative' written on the back of the canvas, which goes beyond the specificity of the title and leaves the viewer with the task of reading the work and interpreting it...

A painting technique such as that of Falco's, which is the result of a passion of execution that is careful and constant, cannot stand being rushed. It reveals itself only through a lingering and thoughtful relationship.

Only in this condition does the plurality of meanings, implicit in the drafting of the images, manifest and reveal itself. It is the response to a slow, meditated and persistent selection of spiritual and poetic consonances."

A light in the chaos,
on the timeline
and you are not alone.
1986

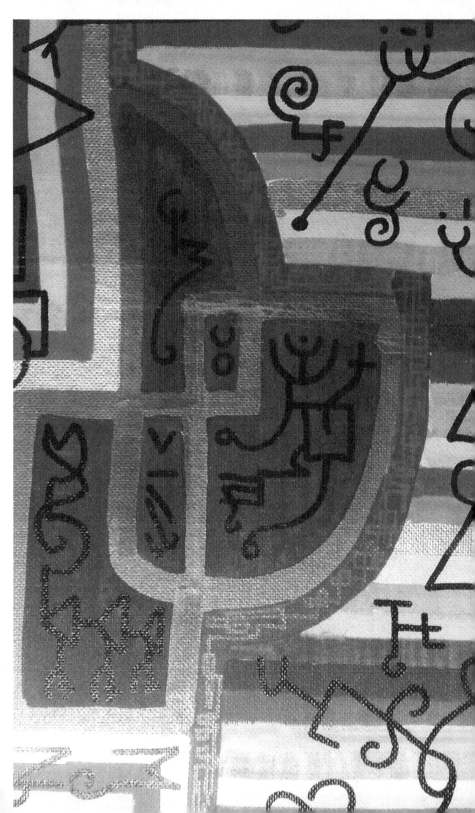

Delfino Mogano, a Damanhurian who is an expert in numerology and astrology, tells about his journey exploring a Selfic painting that is particularly dear to him.

"*In 1985, I saw a painting entitled, 'In the Sign of the Dolphin,' dedicated to one of the animals symbolically linked to the Awakening of the Feminine Divine Forces in our time. For more than two years, Delfino (Dolphin) was the animal name I had chosen as my Damanhurian name, and I didn't hesitate to consider myself as a valid 'representative' of this species. Since then, I have had the painting with me, and it has always kept me company in my bedroom, where over the years, it has welcomed other paintings and Selfic structures.*

What strikes me when I observe it is the sequence of colors in the lines that create the base of the painting. A horizontal sequence has a rhythm of twelve, and the vertical one has a rhythm of four. I've always wondered what their repetition represents, as they also are the only recurrent element in the painting. The other signs that are present, which are in the form of ideogrammatic writing, are all different and seem to be a 'long discourse' that unfolds on different levels.

I sought an explanation for these rhythms through the numbers and the stars. In astrology, there are twelve zodiac signs and four elements (air, fire, earth, water), and they serve as the basis to explain the complexity of the various correspondences between the heavens and the Earth. The threefold repetition of the four elements completes the connection with the twelve astrological signs, each of which 'belongs' to one of the four basic elements that create life.

Observing the painting again, I see that the twelve colored lines seem like a base of musical notes on which the language-signs are elaborated, in a spiraling motion that departs from the center sign— probably 'the sign of the dolphin'—and joins the vertical lines of the four elements, passing onto a different perspective plane.

In this way a 'movement' is created that stretches in a growing, open spiral. In numerology, the spiral is the symbol connected to the number nine, which is an open spiral. It is a frequency-number meaning the connection of various planes of reality, formed by the number eight. Nine draws a spiral-like 'rhythm,' which is the basic form of the energies of the universe as well as that of the majority of Selfic structures."

The creation of Selfic paintings

Knowledge about the creation of Selfic paintings was a prerogative of Falco, so I will let him explain in his own words how they are made. I just added some painting titles to make the text more poetic and evocative.

"Through Selfic painting, I try to give an aesthetic form to my esoteric message. A Selfic painting is a 'living' structure because it interacts with the viewer and the environment, although it is different from the selfs and the personal self. Indeed, there are many categories of forces we can enter into contact with.

The paintings can be considered as 'nests' that are specially designed to attract specific frequencies, so they can contact at least a part of our human world, entering into harmony with the person who will establish a relationship with the painting. The owner of a painting is 'adopted' in turn, because it is indeed a relationship and not a one-way street.

The Selfic paintings—which could also be defined as mandalas or technical signs—bring onto two dimensions a great quantity of elements that are related to other dimensions, where the laws of the universe and forms come together and mix with each other in a different way from that which organizes our space-time."

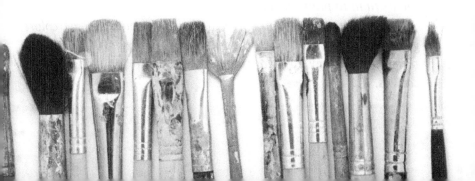

And the Soul,
playing with forms,
caught a reflection of itself
for the first time,
a sliver of color
which we call image
point, line, surface, shape:
it never got out of that fascination
in which it mirrored itself.
1994

"*To get to the point of painting the Selfic paintings, I have followed a fairly complex procedure. First of all, I needed to translate the functions of the metals used in Selfica into colors. I started by personally creating the paper that I used for the paintings and all the colors in a natural way.*

The preparation time was very long. To create pigments used as representations of metals, it takes several years. Later on, it was possible for me to use particularly pure ready-made china inks. Eventually, I built a special Selfic device which I use to prepare the tubes of color that I use for the paintings. In this way, they have the same effectiveness as the pigments I used to make myself.

In this new phase, the value is no longer related to the material with which the color is produced, but rather to the tint itself, that is to its chromatic emission. In any case, the colors I use are always 'treated,' and sometimes it takes longer to alchemically prepare pigments than to paint the pictures.

I use everything from earth to chalks, oil paints, watercolors, glass colors, varnish, mirrors and various materials... I take the function that they have regarding light, and I bring them onto the canvas.

Currently, the main correspondences between colors and metals are as follows: orange is silver, green corresponds to lead, purple and some particular combinations of silver correspond to mica, red corresponds to copper, blue corresponds to iron, and yellow corresponds to gold. White is used to isolate, and black to delineate."

For this painting made of Time,
I use brushes dipped in Duration
and spray a little bit of Future,
I concentrate a few lumps of Past
and melt figures in the Present.
Forms thicken and take on Body,
sounds are recorded together with emotions
and there is also a candle always lit. ...
1992

"I also specially prepare the canvases I paint on with particular liquids that transform them into a sort of parchment that can accommodate several dimensions contemporaneously. A painting represents a two-dimensional projection, but actually it is a cube or a parallelepiped, depending on the shape of the canvas on which it was traced or written. Saying 'drawn', in this context, would not be quite the correct term."

Also two dimensions
have thoughts and mysteries ...
1993

"A Selfic painting has no boundaries. It doesn't finish where the canvas ends, as the canvas is only its focal point in our world. Therefore, before painting, I need to fabricate a 'screen' on which to transfer the images from the channel I want to contact.

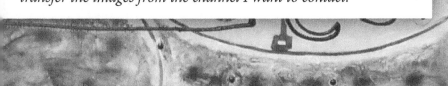

The images that can be received are many and from every field: it is the title that indicates the route for the research. In fact, when I paint, the title usually comes first, or the title and the painting are completed at the same time.

Once the channel is created, all that the positioning of materials and substances which compose the painting do is reproduce what I was looking for."

And here we go,
the written word becomes song,
rhythm, magical sequence of gestures-dance,
power expressed in formulas
that minds, modulating,
can contain and repeat...
So the wise person acquires will,
beyond their tiredness,
inside the energy center previously
located inside every human...
1996

"To the colors and forms in the paintings, I match alchemical, magical and ancestral symbols, and signs and ideograms from what we call "Sacred Language" at Damanhur. The Sacred Language is an ancestral language and the heritage of humankind in many worlds. It is a language that can even allow for communication with forms that are more spiritually advanced than humans.

These symbols activate a correspondence on the deepest levels of the psyche, with the emotional capacities and stratifications of forces present within each one of us. The archetypal signs serve as a key to unlock the room that contains all the answers, the place within everyone of us where knowledge is already fully present."

The letter, and the magical sign,
the word made thought,
identical in the mind of a wise magician
and that of a simple pupil...
so the magic of the brushstroke
hands down an inherent power,
not merely the concatenation
of images-sounds...
Ancestral intuition...
1996

Every sign traced leaves lasting marks...
in the punctiform structure of the Universe...
a gesture gives solid pressures
in the virtual continuum
and the Sole Atom draws
also when it was not born as a form...
but as a pure action.
Magical gesture has no age, nor time...
everything is present and filled with power...
1993

"*When I create Selfic paintings, I use specific systems to spread out the color. These systems are part of the language, and in particular, they give the direction of the reading. There may be layers of color overlapping each other in weaves, diagonally or in other ways. This technique makes it possible to project the meaning of a solid figure, as it determines three directions indicating which dimension is considered in that moment.*

Thanks to the color that is applied with these particular systems, the flat shape of the painting has a different relief in some points. So, the keys of interpretation are based on techniques that use the way of tracing the sign as a reality in and of itself, regardless of the aesthetic result.

Another interesting aspect is the background of the paintings, which can be painted in many different ways. In this case, the direction that is given to the rows of color is important. There are backgrounds that are prepared by making a series of successive lines all in the same direction. There are others which are interwoven with a grid of lines in a horizontal or vertical direction, so as to allow, on different backgrounds, a different flow of the forces in several dimensions, that is, without needing width.

The Selfic paintings are usually created in a very quiet space, so they can welcome the sound that is specifically produced in order to become an integral part of the composition, according to alchemical methods."

And so the written word becomes a song, rhythm,
magical sequence of gestures-dance,
power expressed in formulas that the minds, modulating
know how to contain and repeat...
So the magic of the line handed down
an inherent power,
not only the concatenation of images...
1996

The ensemble of sounds,
the song of instruments and voices,
lights up memories and emotions so ancient
that they connect us to the dawn of humanity,
to the first common matrix of species:
the vital scream, the pulsating heart,
the fast air of the race in the lungs...
2007

"Selfic paintings 'feed' on light because they are sensitive. When I paint parts of the painting in the dark, I use stratifications in such a way that the colors disappear and reappear. As soon as you turn off the light, everything is bright at first, then some parts disappear, then other ones disappear, then they reappear together; some appear first, some appear later.

Because of this, I add different layers, different thicknesses of colors in different points. In this way, the light can emerge little by little, following precise times in its coming to the surface of the canvas. Sometimes I use extremely thin plastic layers with holes made in them, so the color only appears in certain areas and maintains its value when it emerges in successive ones.

For example, there are signs that should be painted white on white. In many cases, I use a color that is identical to the background color, as it is needed for the design.

Sometimes I draw signs on the back of the painting in correspondence with the front part, because they have a value in the transparency. This is a method related to perception, where vision is only one of the senses with which to enter into contact with the use of colors.

The cracks that are sometimes present in the paintings represent the living circulation in various parts of the canvas. Rivers flow within them, and they are the capillary circulation that is expressed with this dilation and contraction of color, so as to create these effects, these lines, these divisions. They are also divisions of potential to create an energetic constriction, a subtle connection. The evolution of a Selfic painting foresees a change, and modification of a two-dimensional object means a transformation of the form; the colors themselves change, as well as their placement.

Of course, the size of the painting is also important because it determines how much space is organized around the painting itself and which uses it may have. Every painting is a door, and the large *ones exponentially increase their functions, but it isn't enough to put together twenty small paintings to obtain what you can do with a large painting.*

In my paintings, another essential element is asymmetry, because if an object were symmetrical, it would repeat itself. Being asymmetrical, it differentiates, becoming a greater variety of things, and it has more depth. This is a way of thinking and, in the paintings, a way to represent the relationship between the object itself and its time, precisely because the object moves and is never the same. Also, it is the relationship between the two-dimensional representation and the three-dimensional subject.

A Selfic painting is really a brush whose function is to draw on the observer to open doors of knowledge, and this is only possible through the exchange and dialogue between the observer and the observed object, through this continuous mirror."

Doors, memories
and transformation

Sometimes, the relationship with the energies of the paintings is so immediate and profound that it triggers fast and significant changes in people's lives. It is as if the paintings were a catalyst that allows memories, talents and new pathways to emerge into the conscious mind, opening new lines of possibilities.

An interesting story is that of Elena Vrublevskaya, a Russian gallery owner, and now also a painter, *"I was one of the sponsors of the Transpersonal Psychology Conference in Moscow in 2010, and I created an extension of my art gallery in the meeting venue.*

For some time, I had been working on a project of displaying art by spiritual teachers or spiritual artists. On the occasion of the Conference, my art gallery in the center of Moscow was hosting a large exhibit of the works of American visionary painter Alex Grey. It was Alex who introduced me to Damanhur and told me I needed to do an exhibit of Falco's art in Moscow.

Esperide came to the conference as a representative of Damanhur, and she brought along two of Falco's Selfic paintings, which I put on display in the Conference venue.

I decided to go visit Damanhur, and I was there one month later. I felt like I had gone back home. I felt a familiarity with the energy, as if it were my native energy. When I saw the Selfic paintings in the Niatel Gallery, it was like a deep remembering of some parts of myself, as if something was reawakening in me. Throughout my life, I have been drawing different symbols in a sort of automatic drawing, and I did not know what they meant. When I saw some of the same signs in the Temples and in Falco's paintings, it felt very strange and also exciting.

I felt inspired to organize an exhibit to share this knowledge with the people of my country, which for me was extraordinary. It was perfectly in line with the mission of my gallery. After six months—and many bureaucratic and logistic difficulties—we opened a wonderful Portal of Selfic energies in the center of Moscow. With the Ambassadors of Damanhur, we created a beautiful event, with seminars, conferences and healing work.

Now, some of the paintings I had in the exhibit have been sold and are in private collections. Some are still with me, and I work with them to meditate and for inspiration. I also like to carry out my activities with them around me. A part of my collection represents the Tarot's Major Arcana, and I also use them to tune in with the different archetypes. My son Darji, who is 12 years old, loves to spend time in the room where I have several paintings. I have noticed that all children love these paintings because they can see the pictures in three phases of light, and this triggers excitement and emotion in them.

Encountering Falco's art opened my own artistic life, which was dormant... I never thought that the symbols coming through me were anything to be taken seriously, then I felt that maybe there was a meaning to this, and I took my drawings more seriously. Now I've had two exhibitions, in Moscow and in Barcelona, and I have even

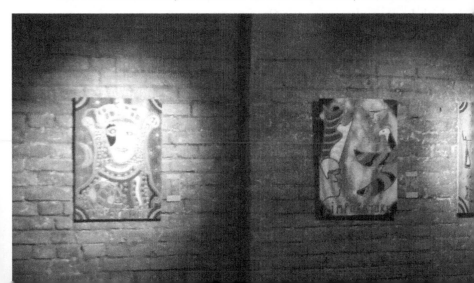

started to sell my work, so now I feel I am really an artist. There are about thirty of my works in private collections—including those of the Princesses of Bhutan. Also, a High Lama from Buthan said that some of the symbols correspond to the spiritual language of the Dakini. This new artistic life gives me a lot of joy and a way to study more about different worlds and civilizations.

Over time, I also acquired a personal self and a spheroself. I do not completely understand what they are, but I feel that this science and these energies are a part of me, maybe from my past. This knowledge is really changing my life and opening an important part of me. I sense that this is just the beginning, and there will be beautiful new surprises in my future!"

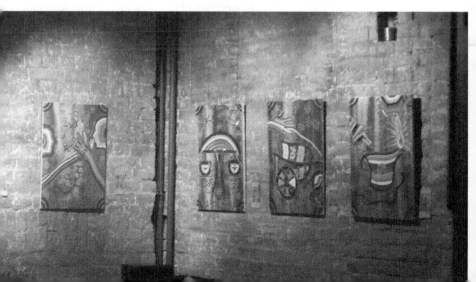

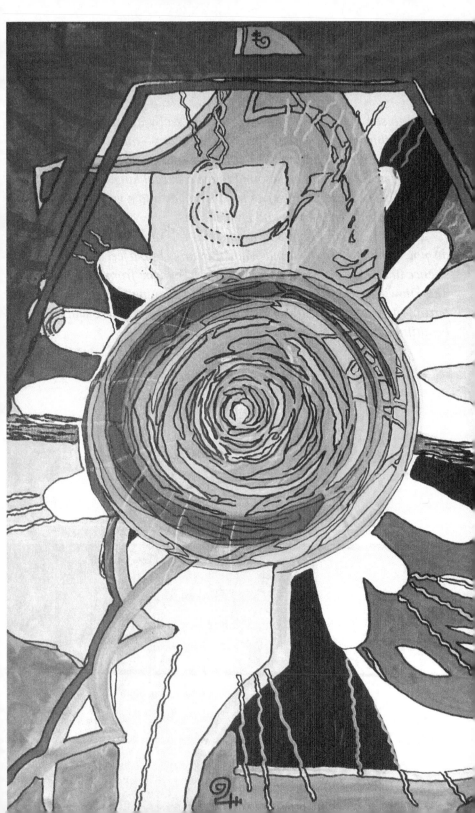

Explorations
in the world of paintings

Over the years, so many experiences of expanded perception have been told by Selfic painting owners. I will share some that offer a taste of the discovery, excitement and satisfaction of being able to open a door of communication with oneself, to be transported into a world of different, more expanded meanings and laws. Often, it can be like a spiritual-psychedelic journey: in a more colorful reality, full of emotions and surprises, a space where thought and form are intertwined, where imagination and perception blend to create worlds of possibilities and new ideas.

Fenice Felce has been a collector of Selfic paintings since the beginning, and he tells us about two very fun experiences.

"One evening I was observing a Selfic painting. Everything was silent around me, and a soft, well-positioned spotlight illuminated the forms, colors and writings of the painting. I was feeling at peace with myself, and I was very relaxed. Suddenly I saw that the painting was moving. It fractioned into many three-dimensional parallelepipeds that were defined in relief, ten centimeters deep! I closed my eyes, but the vision continued as if I had kept them open. So, I opened them and continued to observe this phenomenon.

All of a sudden, a rectangle detached from the painting, pushed by an emerald green flame. It came up to me, struck me in the chest and penetrated right into me. Another rectangle broke away, and again driven by the emerald green flame, it immersed itself into my chest. All the rectangles that were in relief did this. I was so surprised that I lost my breath. In the following two weeks, I realized that my intuition and ability to make connections between various disciplines had notably increased.

Another time, I was in a meditation room at Damanhur, and I decided to sit in meditation staring at the Selfic signs that filled an entire wall, with the intention to discover some meanings about this complex circuit. Experience told me that I would need to stay in contact with the painting for at least twenty minutes. The atmosphere of that sacred space, the scent of the incense, the density of the silence, all makes it so that time passes without you even realizing it; it actually seems to be outside of time. I was sitting still, cross-legged, and I was magnificently well.

All of a sudden, I found myself launched against the painted wall. I was becoming extremely small, and I found myself entering into a point of the Selfic circuit that I had been observing. It was like being in a colored tunnel, like an extremely fast roller coaster. Accelerations, curves, I felt like I was in a very colorful black hole, and I completely lost my sense of orientation. The initial surprise and fear transformed into joy and sheer speed, a desire to see and understand and participate... I was happy, and I let myself be transported in that colorful vortex, full of strange symbols that I didn't understand.

Suddenly, I saw myself getting out, shot out like a cork from golden champagne bubbles. I exited from another point of the painting, far from where I had entered. I found myself dazed and with my head spinning, in my body sitting cross-legged and staring at the large circuit. A truly incredible feeling!"

Another experience that is just as peculiar, which has been repeated over time with many different people present, is that of Eva and Mariapia, longtime friends of Damanhur living in Milan.

"In June of 2010, we were spending some time in the Niatel gallery and several new paintings arrived that were part of the so-called "Geometries" series. We saw two of them that struck us right away and decided to buy them. The paintings arrived to our home

a couple of weeks later, and we placed them in our bedroom next to the other Selfic paintings.

A few months ago, we decided to get a blue laser pen to 'draw on the paintings.' One evening before going to bed, we tested out the laser on the paintings in the dark, as many people do to try communicating with them. We were really surprised when we realized that pointing the light at one of the paintings produced rather unusual optical effects.

When aiming the laser at a black stripe in the center of the painting, a series of reflections were projected onto the ceiling of the room at about a 45-degree angle. They were similar to flashes of light reflected from a pool at night, but there were shapes that followed one another at a speed similar to a Morse code signal. One after the other, a series of symbols seemed to come out of the painting. There were triangles, stars, prisms, parallelepipeds of various shapes, all clearly distinguishable from each other.

While further exploring the painting, we realized that the same phenomenon occurred by aiming the light toward some points in an area that was painted red, just above the black stripe. The signals projected from this area were sharper and more easily distinguishable, because the sequence of projections was slower than the previous one. Upon further exploration, we also discovered that if we aimed the laser without holding it in our hands, a design similar to the painting would slowly appear on the ceiling until it was complete, and then it remained stable.

We successfully repeated this exploration with the blue laser on the painting for many nights.—We also filmed a short video on the phenomenon.—One of the interesting things that we discovered is that the signals appeared weaker and they were harder to read in the nights immediately after periods of absence from our home, as if the relationship with the paintings needed to be nourished by our presence and attention again.

The projection of these figures seems to be a teaching that passes not only through the eyes. Rather, it is a more immersive sensory and emotional experience, bringing to light knowledge that is already in us, just like the title of the painting indicates:

I know how to reignite and reactivate forces and powers,
ancient wisdom and knowledge
contained in you with the goal
of obtaining alchemical substances otherwise lost,
matured by now for centuries and centuries...
2010

For months, during our visits to Damanhur we spent time in the Selfic Paintings Gallery, with the intent of finding other paintings which replicated the phenomenon observed in our geometrical canvas. In November 2012 we finally found one painitng that responded! The title is:

In subtle Selfic connections, I represent paths
that the mind gathers and interprets
to open new spiritual avenues
reaching states which we call "levels of justice."
I join trees and humans,
divine, alchemical and magical connections,
for your own place, in the whole...

That painting had immediately attracted our attention because of a particular three-dimensional effect on the canvas revealed by the black light. We made an attempt with our laser light and... bingo! Pointing the laser on one of the black lines of the design we could immediately see the projection of geometric figures on the painting next to it."

The "Cabin-Gallery"

Several paintings in the same environment connect to each other and create more complex effects than those of a single painting, because they define a space with a precise energetic orientation.

Falco explained that "*a collection of paintings is not just the sum of their number—three paintings together are not just three paintings—rather they are a coordinated structure that can create a series of 'scenes,' a series of interactions of different geometries that transform the space around them. There are paintings that are translations for others; they provide access to the other paintings. It's like putting a key into a lock, and only that key works. Sometimes these keys are formed by the relationship of several paintings that create energetic lines through the subtle bodies of humans and make us more sensitive to what is happening.*

There are 33 key points of energetic access to the energy lines that run through the human body, which are called the 'microlines.' So, there are 33 different angles that indirectly refer to a series of subtle bodies that surround or interpenetrate the physical one.

It's as if each body were a filter, capable of retaining some things and not others. For example, one of them is related to numbers and the primary meaning of numbers. All are specific filters, capable of retaining and giving a function to our energies.

Selfic paintings are prepared with special alchemical substances that act on the microlines. Interaction with a space that is ordered by the presence of at least 33 Selfic paintings—if possible from different periods with different themes and sizes—makes it possible to amplify the microlines themselves. The paintings activate by connecting to each of the filters that compose our subtle structure, which are also related to one or more of our personalities.

So, a basic function of the Selfic paintings is to create and maintain a link among the inner aspects of the individuals who use them. For this to happen, an initial act of will is necessary, expressed through attention in using the painting or Cabin so the Selfic paintings are activated. It is as if observation and light were a ritual act. If the attention on them is continuous, the paintings can stay alive and vital for thousands of years.

If the paintings are adequately combined in the same environment, it is possible to create a system that opens a series of windows within our minds. It also makes it possible to experiment with the 'Threshold,' also during the waking state. The Threshold comprises the different astral planes and the spaces that link the worlds."

An environment with a sufficient number of paintings properly connected to one another is called a "Selfic Cabin" in Damanhurian terminology. This is a space where the vibration of each molecule is modulated to create a constructive interference with the human energy field. The Niatel Gallery, which houses a permanent exhibition of Selfic paintings, is the most complex Cabin in the world, and it is always available for anyone who wishes to use it.

Since the end of 2012, the Niatel Gallery also hosts a newly conceived Selfic structure called "Dimensional Portal." Its function is to widen senses and perceptions. Another Portal is in the Pranoselfica studio and has functions connected to healing and research in the field of health. A third Portal is located near the main stone spiral of Damjl, the capital of the Federation. Its uses are still being investigated.

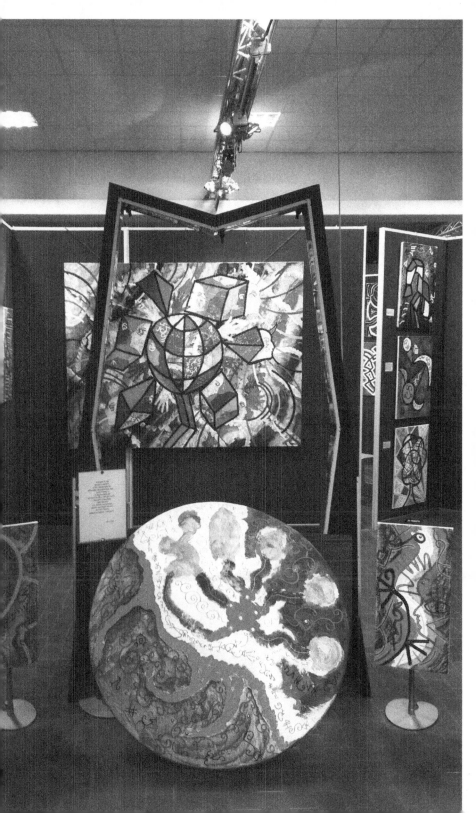

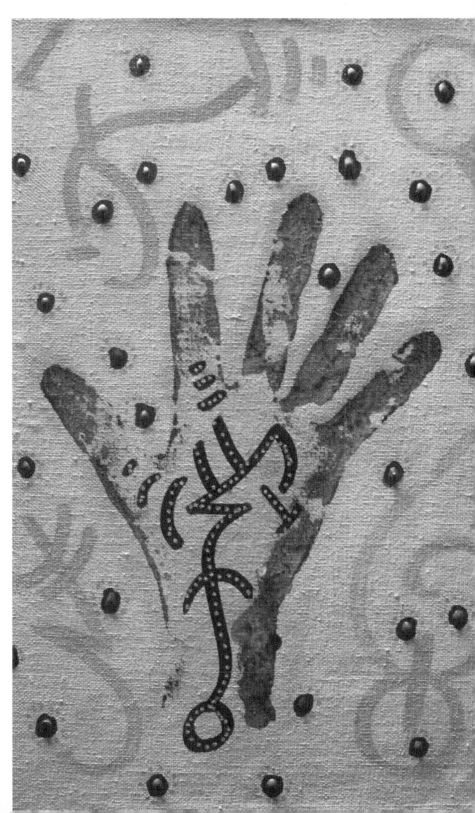

The paintings as "teaching assistants"

The Niatel Cabin-Gallery is used regularly for meditations to prepare for visits to the Temples of Humankind and for special dynamics in some of the courses offered by the Damanhur University. Arciere Aglio, who was already a professional painter before becoming a citizen of Damanhur and is now one of the artists of the Temples, recounts how his relationship with Selfic paintings began during a meditation in his path of becoming a spiritual healer.

"The first time I saw the Selfic paintings of Oberto Airaudi was in 1995 during one of the typical visits and dynamics through which aspiring healers are encouraged to develop their subtle perceptions. After choosing the picture that seemed right for me in that moment, I settled in comfortably and established a visual connection.

With the well-suited lights and music of the Gallery, it didn't take long before I sank first into a neutral state of suspension, then into mild numbness, and finally into a kind of half-sleep with my eyes still open. As I was staring at the signs and colors on the canvas, my mind sailed from one inspired vision to another as if they were dreams. At the same time, waves were moving through me that seemed to be made of loving attention.

The whole experience moved me, and I often wondered about it to myself in the following days, trying to find a placement for that feeling. I tried to understand if those perceptions of mine were due to my particular state of being, to a different way of feeling that morning, or rather to a suggestion or who knows what else.

It would take some time and additional visits to the Gallery to train the appropriate muscles for understanding more, but the emotion revealed itself as a seal of authenticity, proof of something that was very real. That morning, a journey of mutual discovery, attraction and curiosity had begun. It seems to be continuing strongly today, with elements of knowledge that do not come about in a linear way, but rather in a sequence that unfolds according to what I feel, gather, meditate and express; in short, in symbiosis with all that I experience in my life.

During these moments of contact over the years, I have often heard paintings 'calling me' in a loud voice, while others whisper timidly. Other times—for example while experimenting with movement in front of them—I have been 'massaged' with actual physical sensations, and afterward I felt the benefits in my mood and vitality. I have perceived energetic nuclei on the painted surfaces as if they were clusters. I have learned that magic is immense and can be expressed with great power, but it establishes a dialog through 'homeopathic doses.'

I have been tickled, stimulated and teased in more ways than one, especially with intuition. I have had abundant, irrepressible and often euphoric inspirations. I have felt lavished by the flow of energy from the cheerful, bright and silvery frequencies, like giggles that are both childlike and full of complicity.

Thanks to an 'other' kind of refined sensitivity in relation to the Selfic paintings, as an artist in general and specifically as a painter, I have learned to recognize to some extent the 'vitality' that I can express through my artworks. Little by little, I have started to consider my works as living containers that can receive and protectively hold a different quality of energy (in addition to the emanations of my moods). This energy is a kind of... different 'magnetism' that can converse with those who utilize them (and thanks to alchemy studies, all of this is now becoming a personal discipline).

Last but not least, I have always received something from the paintings that could be defined as love, in several forms and gre-

at quantities. Of course it has happened (and still happens) that sometimes I don't feel so much when I am 'too dense' due to the contingent experiences or details of my life.

Or, it could be that trying to rationally unveil the fixed codes that articulate the functioning of the paintings, I have found myself rather bogged down because there is nothing that is very 'fixed' about them (except for a few basic or structural elements and reference points). Selfic paintings are like mirrors that are ready to speak with those who are before them, but we are the ones who activate and animate them with the quality of our presence and the sincerity of our being.

I have studied and written about Selfic paintings for years, and yet I always seem to have an immense, rich and uncharted territory of experiences, perceptions and knowledge before me, ones that—thanks to the paintings—arrive through new and unusual pathways."

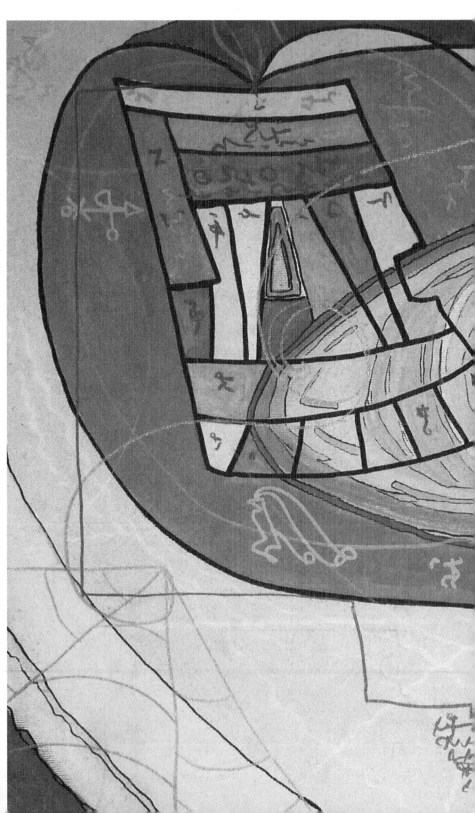

Paintings, life and time

Another use of the Selfic painting Cabin during some of the courses offered by the Damanhur University is completing an operation of "transformation of memories." When in the Gallery, in addition to paying attention to the pictures and using them as an opportunity to train the inner senses, we are also called upon to breathe in the "time scent."

As human beings, we have an internal sense of time that goes beyond the apparent sequence of cause and effect. However, in our habitual way of living and thinking, sometimes events that happed to us when we were children—in which we were not able to choose and make a difference—influence us negatively for years.

Despite the fact that our spiritual and more profound nature does not live in a linear dimension of time, we usually cannot prevent these events from impacting our behavior over the years. If, however, we can change the interpretation that we gave to those events when they occurred, the effects on our present experience can be totally different.

It is not always useful to try and understand, perhaps through years of therapy that unearth painful experiences in all their possible facets, the whys and hows of each event, who has wronged us and when. What is needed is to succeed in writing a different ending to the story, that is, giving an interpretation to the event that transforms the emotional reaction so it has a positive rather than negative effect on us. To do this, one of the systems applied in Damanhur is that of using the potential of interaction between Selfica and our minds, which can guide the creation of a real alternative branch of time with respect to the effects of the chosen event.

This spiritual technology is called "time seeds" because it is applied considering time as a living dimension, similar to vegetation that has several branches and possible directions, which we always have a symbiotic relationship[1] with, just as we have with the plant world.

Echidna tells us that using the Selfic painting Cabin during the course that has the objective of modifying memories has changed some important aspects of her life.

"As I walked amongst the Selfic paintings, I suddenly found myself watching an extremely high-speed movie going backward through the memories of my life. All of a sudden, the scene froze in a small hospital room where I had a CAT scan done when I was eight years old. As an adult, now, I didn't remember what had happened there at all. Before they had me go in, I was waiting in a small hall where relatives were standing and watching the patient on a monitor. On the screen, I saw an elderly woman dressed in all black, lying down and sleeping. Then it was my turn.

Two nurses shifted the weight of the elderly lady who was still there. They put her on a mobile bed that they positioned against the wall a few meters away from me, and they put me in her place, making me lie down in the machine, which was very cold. I was very agitated, and to not waste any time, the nurses strapped down my wrists and ankles with steel bands. To improve the situation, they all left the room and tried to keep me calm by speaking to me with a microphone.

1 According to research in Damanhurian Spiritual Physics, the basic state of matter is not just a wave or particle, but it is also based on "snap time seeds." They make it possible to overcome cause and effect relationships and therefore to create a non-linear response to events. In the manifestation of possible events, there are—temporally speaking—already things that can could happen, and this phenomenon makes a "script" available that can be developed in different ways.

I looked at the woman to my side, and I realized that she was dead... I couldn't stand how they had touched her, ignoring her passage to the Beyond, the confusion, the ridiculous things that they told me to not waste any time with me. I closed my eyes and stiffened up everywhere, keeping my muscles in a spasm.

For thirteen years after that moment, which I had forgotten, I tensed up every time I felt a strong emotional discord. All the times that I felt the laws of the soul were violated, I contracted the muscles of my body, even having to resort to therapists in order to unblock me.

What I realized in that moment as the paintings reawakened this memory in me was that I had absorbed the memory of that discomfort along with the rigor mortis of that woman. I wanted to flee from the painting Cabin, from the hospital room, from my mind. I had a moment of serious emotional confusion. Then I was trustful, and I felt the protection of that prepared place in the company of Selfic intelligences, and I remembered what we intended to do, using the 'time seeds.' I imagined that my story was recorded on film, and I bravely rewound it to the beginning. I found myself lying down again, and instead of closing my eyes and tensing up as they spoke to me and performed my examination, with the knowledge I have now, I guided myself as a child to transform that moment into something better.

I managed to relax, and I sent positive thoughts to that woman. I justified the behavior of the two nurses, thinking to myself that they were probably very tired... and my consciousness of today again consoled that child who was different from the others, comforting her for that pain. Since then, I haven't had any more muscle spasms, and most of all, I feel that I separated myself from that lady, not identifying with her anymore after thirteen years."

The Cabins of Selfic Paintings

In addition to the Cabin created at Damanhur from the permanent exhibition of Selfic paintings, there are other Cabins that have been set up by private owners. Some are for purely personal use, while others are the center of activity for groups of researchers or therapists.

A Cabin has thirty-three Selfic paintings of different sizes, and if possible, from different historical periods, as well as a spheroself that amplifies its functions. Wherever it may be, a Selfic Cabin is a true gateway to higher energies and intelligences, a space for amplifying therapeutic effects and the ideal place to work on perceptions, dreams, and to reach a state of increased integration and mental harmony.

This balance is a fundamental starting point for the blossoming and developing of sensory faculties that are beyond the ordinary, for creativity and intuition in any field you want explore. In this sense, a Selfic painting Cabin is an ideal field for reflection, brainstorming, and planning and designing new endeavors and projects.

It is a spiritual think-tank to turn on all our faculties and connect the functions of the right and left hemispheres of the brain. This happens just by being immersed in the atmosphere generated by the interaction between the vibrational field created by the paintings and that of humans.

At the time that this book is going to press, there are Selfic painting Cabins in Italy, Japan, Croatia, in the United States and in the heart of the Amazon.

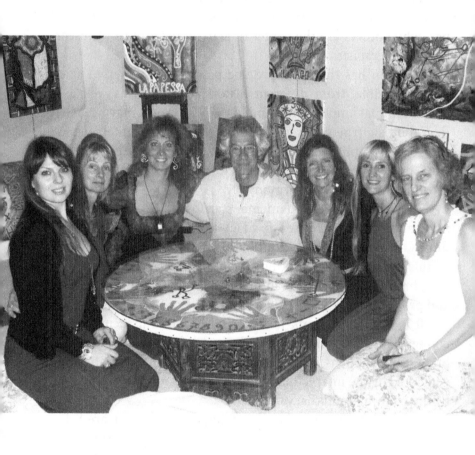

The "Selfic Temple"

In the United States, a Cabin is located in California at Hawks Hill in the Santa Cruz mountains. It is called the "Selfic Temple" by the people who use it, because of the extraordinary quality of the space and the feeling of well-being, peace and self expansion that is experienced inside of it.

Since its inauguration in late May of 2011, this project has been strongly characterized by interaction with the land, especially with the old growth trees present around the house that hosts it, which have become an integral part of the structure. Also, thanks to the presence of an Ouija board painting that can provide indications expressed in language, this Cabin is becoming the heart of a community that meets regularly for meditation and research. Every Full Moon, the Cabin welcomes friends and researchers for a moment of focusing and joyful sharing.

I open the way to unknown worlds,
words that come from the beyond,
where souls, characters and memories are conserved,
personalities and secrets,
stories that are waiting to be told,
to move from anxiety to serenity...
2011

The Cabin is used as a space of amplification for healing with Selfic instruments such as the stiloself and slittino, as well as for massage and energy healing, dreaming and intuition. This experiment is a collaboration with friends of Damanhur and Wisdom University in San Francisco, for the Department of Damanhurian Studies of which Falco was the Chair.

Wendy Grace, the promoter of this initiative, tells how the project of the Cabin took shape.

"*After my first visit to Damanhur in 2000, I did not go back for eight years. I maintained my relationship with the community, and supported their work by producing a book on the Temples with the artists Alex and Allyson Grey. I was surrounded by pictures and the story of the Temple, and a spheroself that I had fallen in love with at Damanhur.*

The possibility opened for me to go back to Damanhur in 2010. When I did, I felt like I reentered a wonderful dream. Since my visit eight years earlier, Damanhur had grown enormously. The outdoor Open Temple, the grounds, the Temples of Humankind all showed the results of years of enormous, dedicated and inspired activity.

During this second trip, I again felt a heightened sense of well-being, and synchronicity seemed to facilitate where I went and what I did. I observed these things, loved them, but didn't really know the depth of the world that supported them. I was at a point in my life to reenter these mysteries, and once again, I felt I wanted to explore Selfica. I finished my trip purchasing another masterpiece of art and technology, a Selfic wand.

A few months later, in Maui, during a meditation in which I was holding my wand, I heard my intuition speak to me inviting me to help facilitate the opening of an energetic portal between Hawaii and Damanhur. I was quite amazed at the suggestion; it did not seem to come from my ordinary mind... So, I decided to create a Selfic Cabin that would connect us in a strong way with the Temples in Italy. I already had about five paintings and a spheroself. I would need 33 paintings in all. When I had about 17, we planned a retreat in Maui to consecrate a portal between Damanhur and Hawaii.

We had commissioned Falco to make a painting to carry the intelligence and energy of the opening. In 2010, we completed the Cabin in California, where I live part of the time, and the work with it has led me to a world and a perception of energy that I could never have dreamed possible.

I am so glad I said 'yes' to the amazing adventure. It has been a challenging and very rewarding journey that continues today. One of the major, secret ingredients to this magic has been the Selfica. So much activity has spawned from my relationship with these intelligences. I have come to know the Selfic energies not from a book or even a lecture but from walking a journey with them. The journey has opened interconnection and memory leading into a greater awareness of community and who I am and who we are in this cosmos, new understandings of time and ways of walking in the world with more peace and joy."

The relationship with intelligent frequencies transmitted by Selfica grows through contact and presence that is cultivated with continuity. The group that inaugurated the Cabin in California has chosen to create a ritualized procedure for activation of the contact, and it has a diary to record presences and impressions.

An interesting comment is that of Rick Buckley: "Taking part in the exploration of the possible functions of the Selfic painting Cabin has deepened my respect and appreciation of the Damanhur technology in helping to bring the spiritual forces back.

The experience has created inside me a new feeling state about being part of the cosmos. I meditate with the new energies I am experiencing in service of the planet. I understand at a deeper level the importance of discipline, respect for the teachings, and repetition to deepen the power of transformation of the separation of earth and spirit."

In the summer of 2013 a second Cabin has been created and activated in Marin County. Connected to the one in Santa Cruz, it represents the "second wheel of an energetic chariot", functioning as a Portal towards very high spiritual forces.

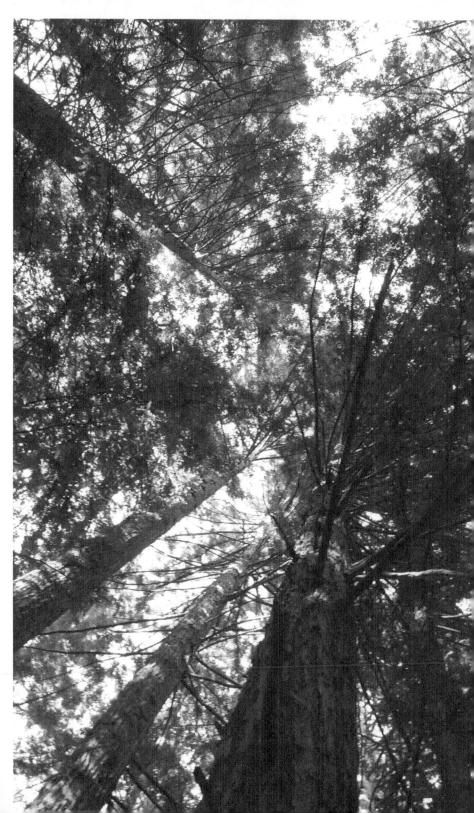

Paintings and forest

The Selfic painting Cabin that is most in contact with nature—and probably the most difficult one to create because of the logistics—is located in the heart of the Brazilian rainforest, 300 kilometers north of Rio Branco. This Selfic structure was created by Robert Wootton, a native of the magical and mystical land of Ireland, who currently lives between Damanhur and the Amazons.

"I bought my first Selfic painting in 2008, because I liked it from an artistic point of view. At that time, I did not understand the significance of Selfica. Then I bought my second and third because they had symbols that had a significance for me; I liked the idea behind the paintings but I was guided to purchase them from a symbolic and artistic point of view. Then I bought a fourth and a fifth, and I sensed that there was something starting to form... I was becoming aware of the energies around them.

I started to go to Damanhur regularly to take courses, and often went to spend time in the Niatel Gallery and started to understand a bit more about it. I heard that it was possible to create a Selfic painting Cabin with thirty-three paintings that could be used to enhance healing and certain faculties explored in different disciplines connected to the Damanhurian teachings.

In the summer of 2010, I reached the number of 14 paintings and was still unsure whether to go to next level. I have been friends with Wendy Grace for some time, and after meeting with her while she was in Damanhur, I discovered that she had approximately 20 paintings and was in the same position as me. I agreed to bring my paintings to her home in California where we combined our paintings to set up a Selfic painting Cabin.

It became apparent what happens when you put them together: the paintings were not separate energies anymore, but they created a container. You look at something that is two-dimensional, but you feel you are in a three dimensional space, and you feel you fall into something that has a completely different, much more expanded energetic quality. The effect of this was initially so strong that we could only spend twenty to thirty minutes in it. Other people came to sit inside the space we had created and could not believe it either... The 'presence' inside the Cabin was truly otherworldly. This experience was the confirmation to complete my own Cabin.

I had been feeling for some time that Damanhur needed to be connected the different ecosystems on the planet, and I now understood how... I left my paintings in California where the messages coming to the group of people who inaugurated Wendy's Cabin confirmed my intuition. They spoke of the need to reconnect to the earth's ecosystem. It was not vague but a concrete requirement for a future path or timeline that we had to connect to.

I returned to the Amazon rainforest, where since 2006, I had been building a Temple, part of which consisted of an eight-sided room on three levels. When I saw the eight-sided space dedicated to the people of the Earth and to the opening onto different worlds and dimensions in the Temples, I knew that that shape had a special significance. This would be the location of the Cabin in the heart of the largest remaining rainforest on the planet.

Over the next year, I ordered some paintings linked to the Tarot that Falco created specifically for me, and I also acquired older paintings, in order to have different types of symbols and a longer 'time span.' I started to take the paintings to the forest, in a journey that required four different flights, five hours by road, half of which unpaved, plus five more hours on a motorized canoe, winding my way up rivers into the heart of the forest, through the dense jungle.

In December 2011, I went back to the forest with the last of the thirty-three paintings and the Cabin was completed, in connection with a spheroself. It is very interesting to experience the presence of *a Cabin in the Forest. The Forest is a very powerful energy in itself. It's so alive that the sensation is not very different to that of being inside a Selfic Cabin. Indeed, there are many similarities between the Forest and the Selfic Cabin. The spirits of nature are so present in the Forest—ditto the Selfica in the Cabin.*

Light has a huge effect on both the Forest and a Cabin. During the daytime, the Forest is very luminous and energized, and there are so many shades of color. At nighttime when you stand under the canopy of the trees, the light from the stars appears to have so many layers; in addition you can sense another form of light that comes from all the living forces that exist there.

In the forest I discovered for the first time that Selfic paintings have a completely different depth and dimension at nighttime. With only natural light present, they appear to have a different energy. They become like starlight and an additional layer manifests... They become something else."

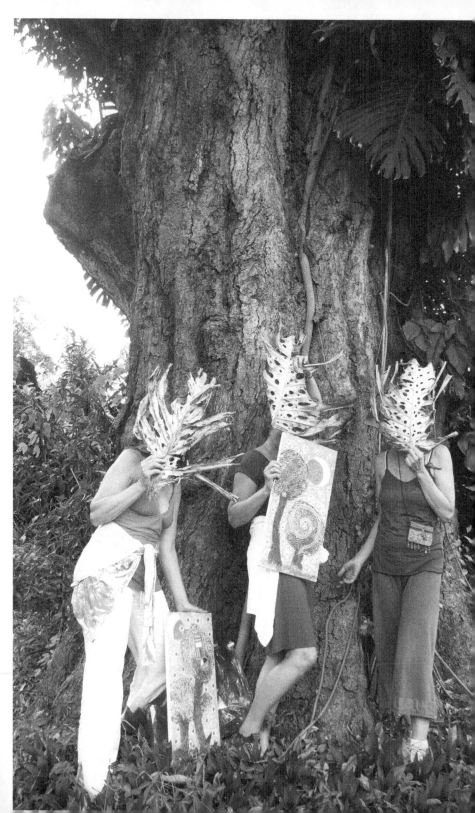

"Alliance with the Pan Kingdom"

When a Cabin of Selfic paintings is kept "alive" by the regular presence of the people who use it, its action extends beyond the physical space where the paintings are located, and it can act as a support for operations involving more extensive contexts. An example of this is the Tree Orientation initiative, which began simultaneously in Japan and California in September of 2011 and then spread around the world.

During the first phases when the Selfic Cabin in California was opened in May of 2011, the researchers there used an Ouija board painting to investigate what might be the most useful functions for this extraordinary instrument that had been assembled there. Communications from the field of intelligence which Selfic paintings give access to spoke clearly and directly about the importance of "feeding on hope" in order to have the strength to continue with one's own task. They indicated a defined field of action: that of our relationship with nature. The messages said, *"Strengthen communication with the trees,"* and *"pledge alliance to the Pan Kingdom"* through *"more actions of joy."*

It was a precise program that referred to a ritual action performed in Damanhur beginning in1989, to connect trees to the protector divinity of planet Earth, indeed Pan, a force that is present again on our plane of existence with his energy, will and knowledge.

Selfic intelligences indicated that it was time to invite every human being to contribute their will and presence in recreating a true alliance between our species and the plant world. This operation would be called "orientation," because the energies and awareness of the trees would be aligned in a common direction, creating a great energetic matrix that puts them completely in communication with each other, even where their roots do not touch anymore. The right Selfic instruments would serve as mediators between the human energies and those of plants, making it possible to foster mutual recognition.

Falco said that one of the objectives was to create a movement of awareness and love of trees through their orientation: an operation that is easy, ritual, peaceful, common, universal, and done without damaging the plant world. In this way, trees could recreate their ancient matrix and, in turn, reawaken human consciousness toward a deeper awareness of the plant world.

Wendy Grace says, "*One of the most significant results of our group's work in the Selfic painting Cabin has been the opening to a new world of trees. Messages we received during our meditations and explorations in the Cabin have guided my friends and me into a deep work with community and with trees and nature.*

The field of energy is vibrant, and nature surrounding the Cabin feels particularly alive. The Cabin has enabled connection with the energy field of the giant Selfic instrument of the Temples of Humankind. It has offered the possibility to connect ourselves and reactivate the rituals and work with trees that Damanhur has been doing for a long time in Italy.

In connection with the Selfic energies, we initiated a project that rapidly spread to places around the world, from Hawaii to Japan, North and South America and all around the world. This work with nature feeds the healthy energy field of the planet. Our actions of orienting the trees, to me, are an act I and others choose to make with the trees, on behalf of all humanity, to compensate for the destruction of 95 percent of the large, giant trees on the planet. Destroying so much of nature, humanity also distances itself from its divine nature.

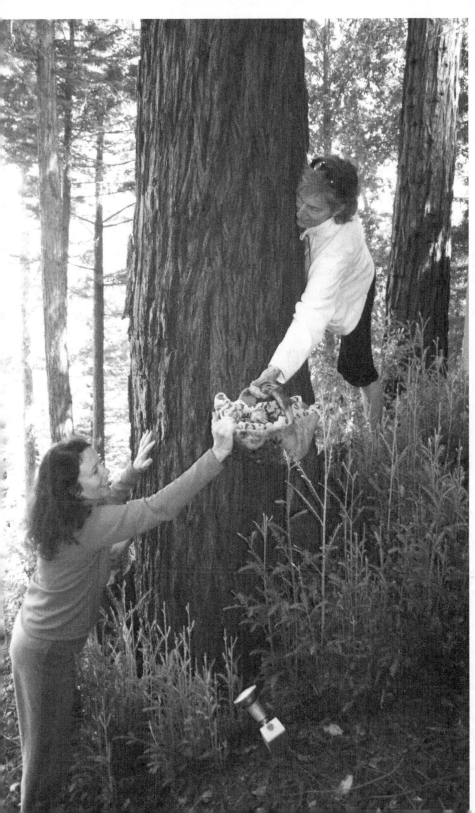

When I circle around the trees with a Selfic instrument, in connection with the Selfic intelligences, a healing begins: the trees return to a purpose they held for the Earth long before humans even walked on this planet. As they heal, they help us restore our relationship with nature and reconnect with our memories so we can know fully once again who we are in the cosmic scheme.

Trees are holders and facilitators of memories. We can walk again in a world where we connect with our divine nature and the sacredness of all life. In the words that came as a prayer for entering the Selfic Cabin and its energies:

We are here to sculpt
a new architecture of being,
awakening community with all beings
and empowering love..."

Harmony with All

Almost at the same time as the orientation in California and Japan was happening, the Amazon rainforest had also become an integral part of the project, thanks to Robert Wootton, who in December of 2011 oriented six thousand trees.

"After completing the Cabin on the third floor of my eight-sided building in the Amazon forest and having placed a Selfic spiral on the second floor directly below the paintings, all was now in place to commence the orientation of the trees in the forest... The first two trees I orientated are two of the most important trees of the Amazon: Castanha the Brazil nut tree and a large samauma.

I then moved away from the building, orienting the trees in a large spiral. Normally you don't leave trails or the path in the forest, as it is dangerous, but to in order to complete my task it was necessary. My objective was to orient 6,000 trees, and I had to walk around each of the first six hundred trees three times. This gave me a complete understanding of how the forest is set up. It is like a cellular system: each giant old tree—a grandmother—has a complete ecosystem around it.

When you look at the forest from the path, you see lines of tree, but when you enter into the dense jungle, you realize that each grandmother supports a family, an ecosystem of other trees, plants, insects, birds and animals.

I had been spending many months in the forest for the previous five years, and I had not understood this—it was like living in a community and not knowing my neighbors. The forest is set up so that each unit repeats itself. It is a mirror of a divine aspect. Moreover, even though the sun is blazing down under the canopy, the temperature is perfect for humans and you walk into the most comfortable environment, full of oxygen. You also realize that everything is reaching for the light, so certain plants are hitching a ride on other plants, and at other levels up high, there are plants that have evolved to live only on air.

I had not put my awareness on all of this and I felt that Selfica was trying to show me something. It lifted the veil more, saying 'look at the structure of everything.' It became obvious that as we perceive, we are transmitters as well as receivers, and we have to learn to receive a bit more rather than just sending out our inner noise.

Selfica reintroduced me to the magic of the plant kingdom, the nature spirits and that there is present all around us beings on many levels or frequencies communicating with us, enlightening us, opening our eyes, so we can realize what is already here.

At a certain point in our human history, we were a part of this community under the trees. Now we have lost the connection to nature, where we evolved from. Now we go to the cities and all we do is to destroy the forest to recreate it with steel and concrete. We need to reconnect... to be in Harmony with All."

A pact
as ancient as life

This joyful, collective, ritual action of orientation to unite the worlds and make peace between humans and "treeness" is needed to re-open a channel of communication with one of the fundamental kingdoms of our planet. Our species has destroyed the connection with this world, not only by destroying the majority of the world's forests, but also through the loss of awareness toward the plant world, which is often considered in the same way as inanimate objects. Taking away the life and spiritual dignity of nature has also deprived us humans of an important part of our soul.[2]

2. According to esoteric tradition, the world we live in was subject to a particular event in the distant past, whose causes are the subject of different theories. This event is supposed to have determined the division of the unitary, integrated primary system. From it, three different worlds originated: the human world, the plant world, and that of the nature spirits. These are the "Mother Worlds," where the divine spark is hosted respectively by humans, plants and nature spirits. Even though these dimensions come from a single matrix, as a result of this division, they are no longer in direct contact with each other. However, they may have an indirect connection through what are defined as "Eco Worlds." Between these three different realities, it is indeed possible to develop a series of intermediate gradations that can contain characteristics originating from more than one of these worlds.

An ancient theory posited by a student of the greek philosopher Cleombrotus affirms that these worlds are located on the vertices of an equilateral triangle, and the various possible eco worlds take form on the respective sides, sixty per side.

The division of worlds does not take place in the whole universe; it has more limited boundaries, although not defined in a precise way. Some ancient myths describe an era in which all the beings belonging to these three worlds coexisted in peace and harmony within the same reality. The nature spirits during that stage of human history were not imaginary beings as they are currently thought of, but they were physical beings just like us. Plant creatures, which today only exist in their specific world, had very different faculties from the ones that trees and plants have now.

Rebuilding this relationship is an indispensable step for reawakening the human species, because it would demonstrate that we are still worthy of carrying the divine spark.

Tree orientation has now involved over one-hundred and fifty millions trees on all continents, and thousands of people connecting to each other through the *"Global Tree Network"* website.

Trees with roots in the water have made it possible to extend this operation to underwater flora. After reaching a sufficient mass of oriented plants in one place, the trees continue on their own, launching the signal and connecting to one another. In Japan, where the members of the Damanhur Center have been particularly active in this objective, at the moment of going to press almost twenty million trees have been oriented.

In this project, a new alliance between the human species and those of plants is the first step in connecting with a greater stellar plan for humanity. The immensity of the project has been illustrated by Falco himself through a series of paintings dedicated to this operation, painted between January and April of 2012.

The division, perhaps due to a natural event or an intervention of external forces, has created a situation that does not allow for the divinization of matter, which can only unfold in a complete and unified reality. A different theory affirms that the golden age does not belong to the past. Rather, it can be in the future that our species and the species of the two other worlds will meet, once the process of the formation of the universe is finally complete.

From "Esoteric Physics," edited by Coyote Cardo, Damanhur School of Meditation Editions, diffusion for internal use, October 2009.

I have always been struck by how this theme is considered with a profound and poetic way in "The Lord of the Rings." The Elves chose exile from our dimension, which is too decayed, and those who remain are destined to fade away, grow old and die like humans. The Ents—tree creatures—are very ancient sentient beings created to protect the trees themselves from lack of respect by humans. The Ents speak, move and choose to join a war alongside humans, but despite the victory, their presence on Earth is destined to fade. Thanks to J.R.R. Tolkien, echoes of this ancient and painful separation between the worlds have touched the hearts of millions, and perhaps it has awakened a little of this ancient memory.

I lead to an ancient alliance,
I orient, choose, balance human and plant forces...

I orient human, powerful minds,
to their natural forgotten task:
the harmony of all, the living whole
that requires the consent of the green species...

I lead thoughts and emotions, dreams,
to the mission that the human species must realize,
a new covenant, a celestial ritual
toward the living plants of our shared world...

The heavenly dream to reconnect the plant world
to the human one, aware,
awakens conscious forces,
capable of liberating, reuniting the planet to the divine whole...
for a cosmic signal which brings humans and plants
on a common planetary path,
happy, aware and evolved...

I lead, orient plant forces to the skies...
By bringing magical temporal vibrations,
I support covenants as old as life,
breathing solstice breaths of history and wisdom, sharing...

I lead the human mind to the agreement with all the herbs
in the world to reach all the way up to the stars...

I orient the plant world, forests, meadows and glades,
living territories to bring back to the alliance
with aware humans,capable of love towards the whole,
the immense skies...

A celestial dance, alive,
to tie and unite ancient brotherhoods
between humans and trees,
with covenants made to reach souls and stars...

There are no skies brighter
than those lit by the awareness of plants,
alive with changes, discoveries and hopes,
oriented by magical human knowledge...

Streets of light with subtle gleams, codified,
bearers of knowledge, of formulas to open the heavens,
reignite stellar flares, talk with the universe again...

Lighted by the moon, the trees start a song,
they begin an ancient dance, millions of years old...
now the song becomes choral
they orient with aware humans...

Connections, encounters, stellar appointments,
to rediscover the mystery, the forgotten, the eternity conquered,
through a concert of happy forests...

The ensemble of different lives makes it possible
to reach extraordinary common objectives.
The ritual guides minds, forces, species
toward the entire galaxy, orienting the universe...

Pulsating like the stars,
the wiser trees observe without commenting:
humans will pass or, guided,
united to the world with us, they will have the stars...

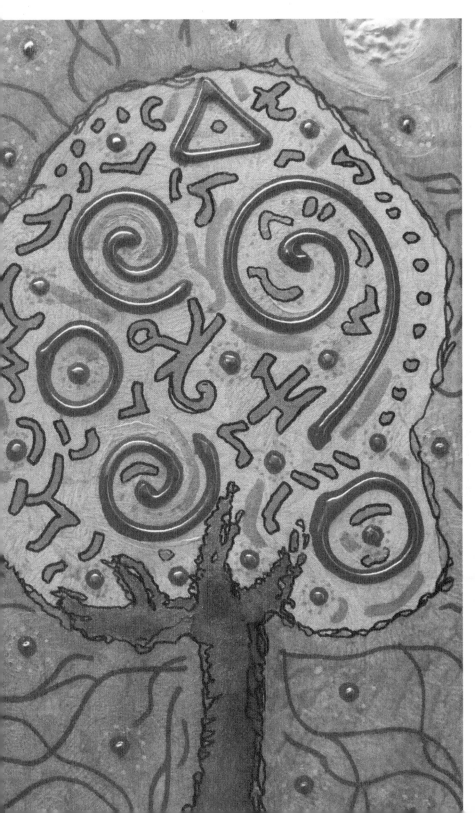

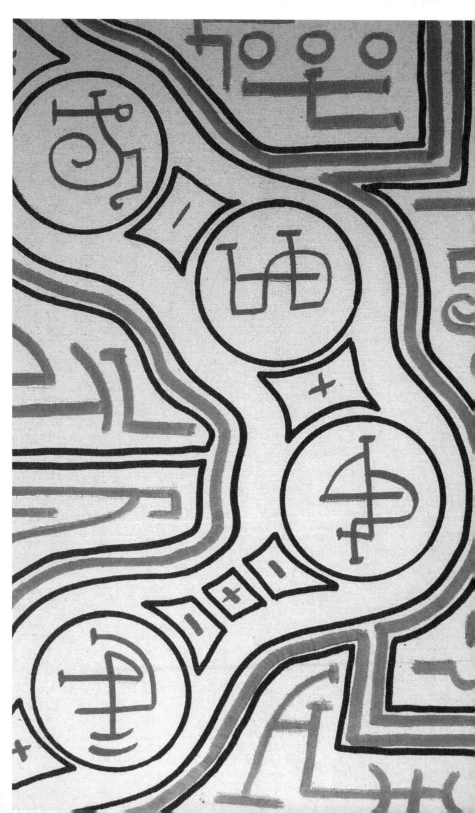

Appendix

SELFICA
Photo gallery
and functions

Most of the experiences described in this book have taken place during seminars and moments of research, but a relationship with the selfs is also a daily affair, an exchange that happens with the Selfic structures that we wear everyday, the ones we have at home, on our walls, in our car. Over the years, thousands of people have bought selfs or given them as as gift, and now there are Selfic structures on all the continents of the world.

Of course, you can enter into contact with all of these selfs and develop a channel of communication through dreaming, intuition and telepathy, or even have a dialog with them. The selfs often respond to an approach that goes beyond a purely functional one. It's worth a try, following your own inclinations. The overall sensation in this research is one of opening new spaces of the mind, in the heart and in our relationships: with ourselves, with others, with life in all its forms.

There are currently about fifty selfs available to the public. The Selfic structures that have microcircuits in them can be prepared to carry out specific functions, by request from the person who will use it.

The SelEt studio, where these selfs are created and produced, is located in the Damanhur Crea center in the town of Vidracco, (TO) Italy. The selfs are also available online at: www.sel-et.com, info@selet.com.

The selfs made in gold and silver are for sale at OroCrea, the jewelers studio also located in the Damanhur Crea, center in the town of Vidracco, Italy (TO). Many creations are available on-line at: www.orocrea.com.

Here are some of the Selfic items that are avaliable. The whole catalogue can be found online: www.sel-et.com.

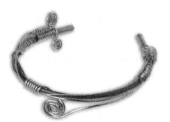

Bracelet for physical well-being. It combines four different functions, to support the body fully: strengthening the vital aura; protection from radioactivity, magnetic, computer and cellphone fields; transforming frequencies of energies that create destructive interferences, and boosting the immune system.

Bracelet for the harmony of mind and emotions, combining three important functions: harmonizing the different components of one's personality, balancing of sensitivity and connecting the mind to the heart.

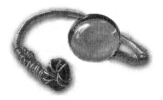

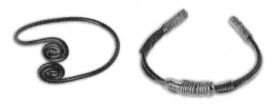

Bracelets for children from birth to 6 years of age, and **for boys and girls** between 7 and 12 years, to support their energy field and help them grow up harmoniously.

Bracelet for creative inspiration, to fine-tune and align the different parts of the wearer's mind, so that inspiration can emerge freely. It can support inspiration in a general way or, with the addition of a micro-circuit in ink, it can be programmed for a specific field, expanding and enhancing the talents already present in the person.

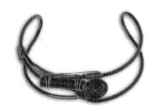

Bracelet for recovering vital energy during sleep. It makes sleep deeper so that four or five hours of rest are sufficient to feel recharged. It is very effective in cases of chronic fatigue and overwork. It is worn around the arm, while sleeping, for up to two or three nights a week.

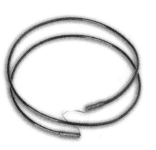

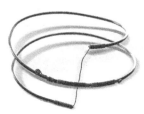

Bracelet to induce sleep in case of insomnia. Its action is most effective if it is worn in the evening for some time before going to bed, but it is useful also if it is put on when waking up in the middle of the night.

Anti-stress bracelet for improving mood, it reduces anxiety and alleviates the problems associated with it. It is to be worn for two hours a day.

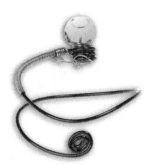

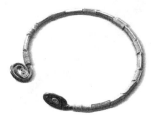

Bracelet for harmonious relationships, first of all with oneself and as a consequence also with others. It supports self-esteem and self-acceptance. It "softens" and harmonizes the aura facilitating the approach with others.

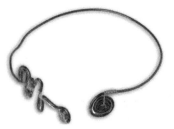

Collar for neck pain. It concentrates its action in the area between the neck and the shoulder blades, producing a general analgesic effect in a very short time. It is to be worn at the onset of pain, with the coils in contact with the nape of the neck, and removed as soon as the aching subsides.

Self to relieve muscle pain and tensions throughout the body. The aching area is to be massaged gently with the glass sphere, turning it counterclockwise for three minutes. The treatment can be repeated every day up to a maximum of four times per day. It can be shared by five people.

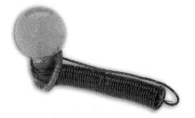

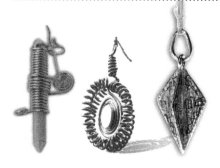

Dowsing pendulums. Thanks to their Selfic part, these pendulums fine-tune easily with the operator, and filter out any expectations that may influence the answers. The one at the center also facilitates contact with the plant world. The third one is made of gold and microcircuits, allowing for complex and highly specialized investigations.

Pen-self: complex Selfic structure applied on a pen. It helps ordering and giving shape to ideas, to receive answers in all fields for oneself and others; it facilitates opening to clairvoyance and automatic writing. Each pen-self is to be prepared with a special activation for the person who will use it. The Selfic structure can be also applied to a pen chosen by the user.

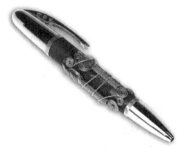

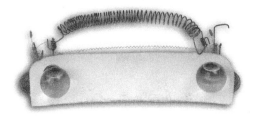

Self to guide dreams. It brings to the surface the most appropriate ones at any time and facilitates their understanding. With additional programs it can be prepared also for cellular rejuvenation during sleep, or as an aid in the treatment of forms of depression.

Self to spread the beneficial effects of the vibration of light and sunshine in any environment, in a radius of about twelve meters around it. Because of its energetic, dynamic and invigorating effects it is recommended for workplaces and homes.

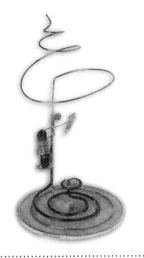

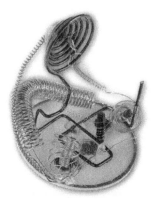

Environmental transformer to harmonize, transform and vitalize the energies present in a specific environment. Prepared on the frequency of one person, it gives the space the "color" of that person. It is very effective for therapists, body workers, energy-healers and councelers, and whenever one's energy footprint is an important part of their profession. It is also useful as a portable "de-charger" for healing or working spaces.

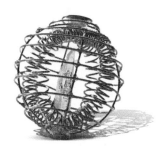

Meditation sphere, to hold in one's hands. It improves focus of thought during meditation.

Damanhur, Federation of Communities

Damanhur is an eco-society based on ethical and spiritual values, awarded by an agency of the United Nations as a model for a sustainable future.

Founded in 1975, the Federation has about 1,000 citizens and extends over 500 hectares of territory throughout Valchiusella and the Alto Canavese area in Italy, at the foothills of the Piedmont Alps.

Damanhur offers courses and events all year round, and it is possible to visit for short periods as well as longer stays for study, vacation or regeneration.

Damanhur promotes a culture of peace and equitable development through solidarity, volunteerism, respect for the environment, art, and social and political engagements.

Damanhur has a Constitution, a complementary currency system, a daily newspaper, a magazine, art studios, a center for research and practice of medicine and science, an open university, and schools for children through middle school. The Federation of Damanhur is also known throughout the world because its citizens have created the Temples of Humankind, an extraordinary underground work of art dedicated to the reawakening of the divine essence in every human being. It is considered by many as the "Eighth Wonder of the World." The art studios that made the Temples are located at Damanhur Crea, a center for innovation, wellness and research, open to the public every day of the year. Damanhur has centers and activities in Italy, Europe, Japan and the United States and collaborates with international organizations engaged in the social, civic and spiritual development of the planet.

Via Pramarzo, 3—10080 Baldissero C.se (TO)—Italy
www.damanhur.org

CPSIA information can be obtained at www.ICGtesting.com
Printed in the USA
BVOW08s1922220614

356955BV00027B/588/P